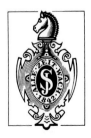

P. Beighton   B. J. Cremin

Sclerosing Bone Dysplasias

Foreword by H. G. Jacobson

62 Figures containing 218 Illustrations

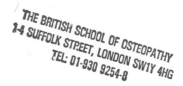
Springer-Verlag
Berlin Heidelberg New York 1980

Professor Peter Beighton, M.D., Ph.D., F.R.C.P., D.C.H.
Department of Human Genetics,
Medical School and Groote Schuur Hospital,
University of Cape Town,
South Africa

Professor Bryan J. Cremin, F.R.A.C.R., F.R.C.R.
Department of Radiology,
Groote Schuur and Red Cross Children's Hospital,
University of Cape Town,
South Africa

ISBN 3-540-09471-7 Springer-Verlag Berlin Heidelberg New York
ISBN 0-387-09471-7 Springer-Verlag New York Heidelberg Berlin

Library of Congress Cataloging in Publication Data. Beighton, Peter. Sclerosing bone dysplasias.
Bibliography: p. Includes index. 1. Osteosclerosis—Atlases. 2. Bones—Abnormalities—Atlases.
3. Bones—Radiography—Atlases. I. Cremin, Bryan Joseph, joint author. II. Title.
RC931.08B44   616.7′1   79-24616   ISBN 0-387-09471-7

© by Springer-Verlag Berlin Heidelberg 1980
Printed in Germany.

Printing and bookbinding: Brühlsche Universitätsdruckerei, Giessen
2128/3140-543210

To Greta and Sybil

Foreword

Much confusion exists in the accurate identification and classification of the many disorders in infancy which affect the skeleton by producing sclerosing lesions throughout the entire skeleton or in selected areas. A scholarly effort to bring order into this confusing field must be welcomed.

Professors Beighton and Cremin have skillfully defined the problem and concisely yet thoroughly have identified the various sclerosing dysplasias. They bring to this task a wealth of clinical experience in their many years in the Departments of Radiology at the University of Cape Town Medical School and the Groote Schuur and Red Cross Children's Hospitals in Cape Town, South Africa. The authors also have had available data from the University of Cape Town Skeletal Dysplasia Registry.

Professors Beighton and Cremin have used as a basis for their treatise the Paris Nomenclature (the modified version of 1977). This monograph is a felicitous combination of a working atlas and a scholarly exposition of the various sclerosing bone dysplasias, considering in detail eighteen major entities adopted from the Paris classification. Other disorders which present with osteosclerosis are also described. These include Caffey disease, oculodento-osseous dysplasia, central osteosclerosis with bamboo hair, fluorosis, osteosclerosis associated with renal disease and mastocytosis.

Each of the eighteen bone dysplasias is discussed in a very well organized format. Each entity includes as an introduction a section on historical-nosological considerations, followed by a description of the clinical features. The radiological findings are emphasized, using a systematic approach. A section on general comments is incorporated. A concise but relevant bibliography is included for each of the sclerosing dysplasias and at the end of each section a radiological atlas of the cases encountered is presented.

This monograph should serve as a welcome contribution for a variety of physicians. Radiologists, and particularly pediatric and skeletal radiologists, will find this work a storehouse of information. The clinical pediatrician and orthopaedic clinician too, will be similarly rewarded. The medical geneticist will find the data presented of great interest.

Residents in training in radiology, pediatrics and orthopaedics as well as medical students should welcome such a work in helping to identify a complex group of disorders. The treatise is concisely written with admirable clarity and the illustrations themselves should virtually characterize for the reader each of the disorders described. The text makes for enjoyable reading and the scope of the book should establish it as an important reference source.

February, 1980   HAROLD G. JACOBSON, M.D.

Acknowledgements

We are greatly indebted to:

Mrs THELMA HOCHSCHILD, Chief Radiographer at the Red Cross
Children's Hospital, Cape Town, for undertaking the major task of
organising the illustrative material and bringing order out of chaos:
without her assistance this book would never have been finished in time.
Professor HERMAN HAMERSMA, of the Department of
Otorhinolaryngology, University of Pretoria, for his collaboration in the
investigation of patients and for provision of case material.
Colleagues who provided radiographs and journal editors for their
permission for published illustrations to be reproduced. Individual
mention is given and references cited in the relevant chapters.
The secretaries GILLIAN SHAPLEY, BARBARA BREYTENBACH, JANET
GROOM and BERRY NEUMANN, who typed the manuscript with
enthusiasm and dedication.
Mrs SUE HENDERSON for her skill and patience in the preparation of
photographs.
The nursing sisters in the Department of Human Genetics, Mrs
R. DUGGAN and Miss M. MACRAE for their assistance in assembling the
clinical and radiographic data.
Dr H. S. MYERS of Cape Town for his perceptive and constructive
criticism of the embryo manuscript and for his valuable comments
during the final stages.
The South African Medical Research Council and the University of
Cape Town Staff Research Fund for their support of our investigations.

Cape Town, January, 1980   PETER BEIGHTON
                                            BRYAN J. CREMIN

Table of Contents

Introduction

The sclerosing bone dysplasias are characterised by varying degrees of increased skeletal density and abnormal modelling. Osteopetrosis, or ALBERS-SCHÖNBERG disease, is the prototype and best known of these disorders but many others have now been delineated. They differ in their course, prognosis and genetic background, and for this reason diagnostic precision is crucial. In the majority, this is achieved by recognition of the characteristic radiographic manifestations and consequently the radiologist plays a key role in the management of patients with these conditions.

Much of the confusion surrounding the sclerosing bone dysplasias has arisen because of semantic problems. In order to clarify this situation we have given a brief account of the development of concepts and terminology concerning each condition, and where appropriate, alternative names have been tabulated. Many of the references were obtained following a computerised information retrieval search and they have been selected on the basis of topicality, comprehensiveness or because they are of historical importance.

The general outline of the contents follows the 1977 Paris Nomenclature, but we have based designations upon popular usage, and in accordance with modern practice, the possessive form of eponyms has been avoided. Chapter length is related to the clinical importance and current interest, and in some instances, information concerning every case in the literature has been listed.

In the radiological sections we have employed a systematic approach, dividing the skeleton into four definite regions. The abnormal findings have been described in this way to provide the radiologist with both a method of examining radiographs and an easy form of reference. The illustrations follow the text in every chapter, and for completeness the figure legends have been used to supplement our radiological comments. Only a few radiologists make skeletal dysplasias their speciality, and the remainder will find it impossible to commit facts to memory unless they are reinforced by actually seeing the patient. It may be only then that a piece of the puzzle is remembered and put into place. A blanket diagnosis of some form of 'osteopetrosis' is no longer sufficient, but the temptation to force the facts into a syndrome which they do not fit must be resisted. A philosophy of radiographic evaluation is provided in Chap. 3.

This book is intended to serve as a reference atlas or compendium for radiologists, but it contains information which will be of interest to orthopaedic surgeons, medical geneticists, and paediatricians. We have written this work in the light of our own experience of sclerosing bone dysplasias, using data in the University of Cape Town (Department, 57 Human Genetics) Skeletal Dysplasia Registry. The majority of illustrations are derived from this collection, although in certain rare conditions overseas colleagues have kindly provided material. The sources are acknowledged at the end of each chapter.

Chapter 1

History and Nomenclature

The recent history of the sclerosing bone dysplasias began in Germany when ALBERS-SCHÖNBERG (1904) published 'roentgenograms of a rare bone disease' concerning a young man with increased density of the skeleton. Sporadic reports followed and the term 'osteopetrosis' or 'stony bones' came into general use. During the next quarter of a century, osteopoikilosis (LEDOUX-LEBARD et al. 1916), melorheostosis (LÉRI and JOANNI 1922), osteopathia striata (VOORHOEVE 1924; FAIRBANK 1925), and diaphyseal dysplasia (CAMURATI 1922; ENGELMANN 1929) were all delineated. Many patients with 'atypical' osteopetrosis were reported and it later became apparent that this designation encompassed numerous distinct disease entities. In the same period, facial distortion by bone overgrowth was often labelled 'leontiasis ossea.' Retrospectively, firm diagnoses of specific sclerosing bone dysplasias can be made in a number of individuals who had previously been grouped in these general categories.

Craniometaphyseal dysplasia and Pyle disease were differentiated by JACKSON et al. (1954) and the observations of these investigators were confirmed by GORLIN et al. (1970). During the same period BAKWIN and EIGER (1956) described the condition currently known as 'osteoectasia with hyperphosphatasia,' while TRUSWELL (1958) encountered 'osteopetrosis with syndactyly,' now termed 'sclerosteosis.' Other disorders delineated in this era include craniodiaphyseal dysplasia (JOSEPH et al. 1958), pycnodysostosis (MAROTEAUX and LAMY 1962), osteodysplasty (MELNICK and NEEDLES 1966), dysosteosclerosis (SPRANGER et al. 1968), and frontometaphyseal dysplasia (GORLIN and COHEN 1969). Further heterogeneity has been recognised in several of these conditions, and in the majority, the genetic background has been determined.

The sclerosing bone dysplasias were discussed in the 1951 edition of Sir Thomas Fairbank's *Atlas of General Affections of the Skeleton* and they were reviewed by RUBIN (1964) in his *Dynamic Classification of Bone Dysplasias*. A significant advance in understanding took place when GORLIN et al. (1969) published their critical analysis of genetic craniotubular dysplasias and hyperostoses. Subsequently, conditions in these groups were extensively reviewed in an edition of *Progress in Paediatric Radiology* devoted to intrinsic diseases of bones (KAUFMANN 1973), and their features were depicted by SPRANGER et al. (1974) in Bone Dysplasias: An *Atlas of Constitutional Disorders of Skeletal Development*.

In 1969 a group of experts convened by Dr PIERRE MAROTEAUX met in Paris under the aegis of the European Society of Paediatric Radiologists and formulated a nomenclature for constitutional diseases of bone. Their primary purpose was to unify the terminology at an international level and they emphasised that they had not attempted to produce a classification of bone disorders. The sclerosing bone dysplasias were listed in the Paris Nomenclature under the subheading 'abnormalities of density, of cortical diaphyseal structure or metaphyseal modelling or both' (MAROTEAUX 1970). The Nomenclature was updated in 1977, and the revised version of the relevant sub-section is given below:

Osteopetrosis with precocious manifestations
Osteopetrosis with delayed manifestations (several forms)
Pycnodysostosis
Osteopoikilosis
Osteopathia striata
Melorheostosis
Diaphyseal dysplasia, CAMURATI-ENGELMANN
Craniodiaphyseal dysplasia
Endosteal hyperostosis
   a) Autosomal dominant, WORTH
   b) Autosomal recessive, VAN BUCHEM
Tubular stenosis, KENNY-CAFFEY
Pachydermoperiostosis
Osteodysplasty, MELNICK-NEEDLES
Frontometaphyseal dysplasia
Craniometaphyseal dysplasia (several forms)
Metaphyseal dysplasia, PYLE
Sclerosteosis
Dysosteosclerosis
Osteoectasia with hyperphosphatasia.

References

ALBERS-SCHÖNBERG H (1904) Röntgenbilder einer seltenen Knochenerkrankung. Münch Med Wochensch 51:365
BAKWIN H, EIGER MS (1956) Fragile bones and macrocranium. J Pediatr 49:558
CAMURATI M (1922) Di un raro caso di osteite simmetrica creditatia degli arti inferior. Chir Organi 6:662
ENGELMANN G (1929) Ein Fall von Osteopathia Hyperostica (sclerotisans) Multiplex Infantalis. Fortschr Roentgenstr 39:1101
FAIRBANK HAT (1925) A case of unilateral affection of the skeleton of unknown origin. Br J Snrg 12:594
FAIRBANK HAT (1951) An atlas of general affection of the skeleton. Livingstone, Edinburgh, p 32
GORLIN RJ, COHEN MM (1969) Frontometaphyseal dysplasia. Am J Dis Child 118:487

GORLIN RJ, SPRANGER J, KOSZALKA MF (1969) Genetic craniotubular bone dysplasias and hyperostoses. A critical analysis. Birth Defects V (4):79

GORLIN RJ, KOSZALKA MF, SPRANGER J (1970) Pyle's disease (Familial Metaphyseal Dysplasia). J Bone Joint Surg [Am] 52:347

JACKSON WPU, ALBRIGHT F, DREWRY G, HANELIN J, RUBIN MI (1954) Metaphyseal dysplasia, epiphyseal dysplasia, diaphyseal dysplasia and related conditions. Arch Intern Med 94:871

JOSEPH R, LEFEBVRE J, GUY E, JOB JC (1958) Dysplasia cranio-diaphysaire progressive. Ses relations avec la dysplasia diaphysaire progressive Camurati-Engelmann. Ann Radio (Paris) 1:477

KAUFMANN HJ (ed) (1973) Intrinsic diseases of bones. Karger, Basel (Progress in pediatric radiology, vol 4)

LEDOUX-LEBARD R, CHABANIX, DESANNE (1916) L'osteopoecilie, form nouvelle d'osteite condensante generalisée. J Radiol Electrol Med Nucl 2:133

LÉRI A, JOANNI J (1922) Une affection non décrite des os: hyperostose 'en coulée' sur toute la langueur d'un membre où mélorhéostose. Bull Soc Méd Hôp Paris 46:1141

MAROTEAUX P (1970) Nomenclature internationale des maladies osseuses constitutionelles. Ann Radiol (Paris) 13:455

MAROTEAUX P, LAMY M (1962) La pycnodysostose. Presse Méd 70:999

MELNICK JC, NEEDLES CF (1966) An undiagnosed bone dysplasia: A 2 family study of 4 generations and 3 generations. A J R 97:39

RUBIN P (1964) Dynamic classification of bone dysplasias. Year Book Medical Publishers, Chicago, p 258

SPRANGER J, ALBRECHT C, ROHWEDDER H-J, WIEDEMANN H-R (1968) Die Dysosteosklerose: eine Sonderform der generalisierten Osteosklerose. Fortschr Roentgenstr 109:504

SPRANGER J, LANGER LO, WIEDEMANN HR (1974) Bone dysplasias. An atlas of constitutional disorders of skeletal development. Saunders, Philadelphia

TRUSWELL AS (1958) Osteopetrosis with syndactyly. A morphological variant of Albers-Schönberg disease. J Bone Joint Surg [Br] 40:208

VOORHOEVE N (1924) L'image radiologique non encore décrite d'une anomalie du squelette. Acta Radiol (Stockh) 3:407

Chapter 2

Clinical and Genetic Aspects

The sclerosing bone dysplasias are all uncommon and some are distinctly rare. In order to give a perspective of their relative prevalence, the approximate totals of reported cases in the world literature and their modes of inheritance are given in Table 2-1.

Complications and Prognosis

The sclerosing bone dysplasias vary greatly in their prognosis and some, such as sclerosteosis and dysosteosclerosis, are potentially lethal. Others, including Pyle disease and the dominant form of osteopetrosis, cause only minor clinical problems, while at the other end of the spectrum, osteopoi-

Table 2-1. Sclerosing bone dysplasias – Prevalence and mode of inheritance

	Published cases	Genetic background
Osteopetrosis with precocious manifestations	50	AR
Osteopetrosis with delayed manifestations	500	AD (Heterogeneous)
Pycnodysostosis	100	AR
Metaphyseal dysplasia (PYLE)	20	AR
Craniometaphyseal dysplasia	50	AD/AR
Craniodiaphyseal dysplasia	10	AR
Frontometaphyseal dysplasia	15	XL?
Osteodysplasty (MELNICK-NEEDLES)	25	AD
Dysosteosclerosis	12	XL
Endosteal hyperostosis: (i) AD type – WORTH	35	AD
(ii) AR type – VAN BUCHEM	15	AR
Sclerosteosis	50	AR
Diaphyseal dysplasia (CAMURATI-ENGELMANN)	100	AD
Osteopathia striata	100	AD
Osteopoikilosis	300	AD
Melorheostosis	250	–
Osteoectasia with hyperphosphatasia	30	AR
Infantile cortical hyperostosis (CAFFEY)	400	?
Oculodento-osseous dysplasia	65	AD/AR?

Key: AD = Autosomal dominant.
AR = Autosomal recessive.
XL = X-linked.

kilosis is clinically silent. There is diversity in the course of these conditions. For instance osteoectasia and craniodiaphyseal dysplasia are progressive, while infantile cortical hyperostosis and CAMURATI-ENGELMANN disease tend to regress. Complications, such as bone fragility, as in pycnodysostosis, or a propensity to cranial nerve compression, as in craniometaphyseal dysplasia, are fairly consistent in any particular disorder. For these reasons, accurate diagnosis is important for rational prognostication.

Management

Surgical intervention plays an important role in the management of these dysplasias, and relief of bony entrapment of cranial nerves and prophylactic craniotomy to lower intracranial pressure are often of value. Specialised dental care, including removal of impacted teeth and the correction of malocclusion or mandibular prognathism, may be indicated. From the orthopaedic point of view, treatment centres around pathological fractures and secondary deformities. All surgical procedures are influenced by the abnormal consistency and thickness of the skeleton.

At the present time there is no specific medicinal therapy, but drugs such as calcitonin and diphosphonates may eventually prove efficacious in some of these conditions (WHALEN et al. 1977).

Basic Defect

The basic structural defect is unknown in the sclerosing bone dysplasias, and with few exceptions, biochemical studies yield unremarkable results, while the chromosomes are normal in each of these disorders. However, specific histological changes that may throw light on the underlying disease mechanisms are beginning to be reported (KAITILA and RIMOIN 1976). The pathogenesis of osteopetrosis has been studied by many researchers (RAGAB et al. 1975) and animal models are available (MARKS 1978). New techniques such as bone-mineral analysis by ion activation hold promise for the future.

Genetics

Information concerning the genetic background of any condition is crucial for the assessment of recurrence risks. Virtually all the sclerosing bone dysplasias are inherited and relevant genetic data are mentioned in the text. A review of the various mechanisms of inheritance is outside the scope of this book, but it is assumed that the reader is aware of the different implications of dominant and recessive transmission. By way of example, a pedigree showing autosomal dominant inheritance of craniometaphyseal dysplasia is given in Fig. 2-2, while autosomal recessive transmission of Pyle disease is shown in the family tree in Fig. 2-1.

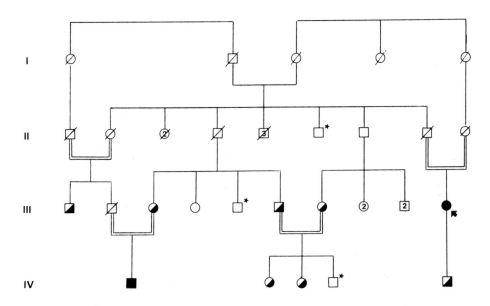

Fig. 2-1. The pedigree of a family with Pyle disease. The parents of the affected male and female were normal but consanguineous. Several obligatory or potential heterozygous carriers of the abnormal gene had minor degrees of femoral metaphyseal widening (Raad and Beighton 1978)

Key to Pedigree

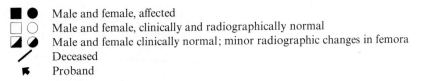

■ ●   Male and female, affected
☐ ○   Male and female, clinically and radiographically normal
◪ ◗   Male and female clinically normal; minor radiographic changes in femora
/   Deceased
◤   Proband

The detection of clinically asymptomatic heterozygous carriers of the abnormal gene in autosomal recessive disorders is important from the point of view of genetic counselling and prevention. Minor radiographic changes are probably present in 'carriers' in sclerosteosis and Pyle disease (see Chap. 6, Fig. 6-13a). New radiographic techniques, such as photon absorptiometry for the objective measurement of bone density or thickness, may prove to be of value in this situation.

There is little doubt that many of these conditions are heterogeneous. This has already proved to be the situation in endosteal hyperostosis (Worth and van Buchem types), and evidence is accumulating to indicate that there are several distinct forms of osteopetrosis. It is to be anticipated that the recognition of specific metabolic or structural defects will permit some sclerosing dysplasias to be split into separate entities. In turn, this delineation will form the basis for the formulation of optimal regimes of management.

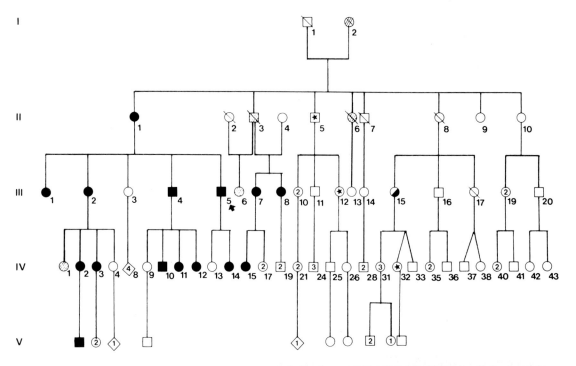

Fig. 2-2. The pedigree of a kindred with the
autosomal dominant form of craniometaphyseal
dysplasia. In this type of inheritance, the
condition is transmitted from generation to
generation. Any child of an affected person has
an even chance of receiving the abnormal gene
and thus developing the disorder (Beighton
et al., 1979)

Key to Pedigree

■ ● Affected male and female
◣ ◖ Affected male and female – deceased
▨ ▨ Thought to be affected – not seen
▨ ▨ Thought to be affected – deceased
☆ ★ Hearing problems
◤ ◑ Facial paralysis
⊠ ⊘ Unaffected male and female – deceased
□ ○ Unaffected male and female
🢥 Proband

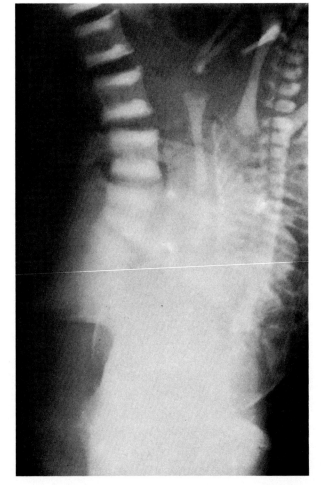

Fig. 2-3. Osteopetrosis in a mother and fetus
detected by chance during radiographic
pelvimetry (Delahaye et al. 1976)

Antenatal Diagnosis

At the present time none of the sclerosing bone dysplasias are amenable to antenatal diagnosis in early pregnancy, although the autosomal dominant form of osteopetrosis has been recognised by chance in late pregnancy (Fig. 2-3). However, genetic knowledge is increasing rapidly and it is possible that the recognition of these conditions in the fetus will eventually be feasible. In this context, the recurring theme of diagnostic precision arises, as decisions concerning the monitoring of a pregnancy and possible therapeutic termination are based upon clinical prognosis and the genetic recurrence risks.

Distribution

The ethnic and geographical distribution of the sclerosing bone dysplasias is apparently very uneven. This is partly a reflection of the availability of radiographic facilities and diagnostic sophistication, but is also the result of historical accidents and biological pressures that have influenced the population frequencies of the abnormal genes. The high prevalence of osteoectasia with hyperphosphatasia in persons of Costa Rican stock or the virtual limitation of sclerosteosis to the Afrikaner community of South Africa exemplify this situation. These facts are of importance in the process of differential diagnosis, and for this reason information of this nature is given in the appropriate chapters.

References

BEIGHTON P, HAMERSMA H, HORAN F (1979) Craniometaphyseal dysplasia – variability of expression within a large family. Clin Genet 15:252

DELAHAYE RP, METGES PJ, ANGLADE JP, MALMEZAT X, PASCAL-SUISSE P (1976) Découverte simultanée d'une ostéopétrose chez la mère et le foetus à l'occasion d'une radiopelvimétrie. J Radiol Electrol Med Nucl 57/4, 359

KAITILA I, RIMOIN DL (1976) Histologic heterogeneity in the hyperostotic bone dysplasias. Birth Defects 12/6:71

MARKS SC (1978) Studies of the mechanism of spleen cell cure for osteopetrosis in 'ia' rats: Appearance of osteoclasts with ruffled borders. Am J Anat 151:119

RAAD MS, BEIGHTON P (1978) Autosomal recessive inheritance of metaphyseal dysplasia (Pyle). Clin Genet 14:251

RAGAB AH, DUCOS R, CRIST W, DUCK SC (1975) Granulopoiesis in osteopetrosis. J Pediatr. 87:422

WHALEN JP, HORWITH M, KROOK L, MACINTYRE L, MENA E, VITERI F, TORUN B, NUNEZ EA (1977) Calcitonin treatment in hereditary bone dysplasia with hyperphosphatasemia: A radiographic and histologic study of bone. A J R 129:29

Chapter 3

Radiological Considerations

Semantic and diagnostic confusion concerning sclerosing bone dysplasias poses special problems for radiologists. This difficulty was brought forcefully to our attention when one of our first patients presented with a familial skeletal disorder which had been labelled at various times as 'Albers-Schönberg disease', 'marble bones', 'osteopetrosis', 'leontiasis ossea' and 'Pyle disease'. Following clinical and radiographic investigations, it became evident that he had the autosomal dominant form of craniometaphyseal dysplasia.

Radiological Evaluation and Techniques

The technique of radiological evaluation is standard in many institutions, but the following points are of importance:

a) The radiographic changes in the sclerosing bone dysplasias are age-related, and on occasion it may be necessary to await the development of the syndrome before a diagnosis can be reached. Equally, a radiologist is often given radiographs only of the limbs of a bone dysplasia patient for identification. He must, however, view the whole skeleton before giving a definitive answer.

b) In patients with a recognisable disorder, radiographic survey should consist of at least one view of each bony region. It is our practice to make an initial 'scout survey' which consists of at least the following seven basic films:

Skull, lateral

Thoracic and lumbar spine, lateral (2 films)

Chest and shoulders, PA

Pelvis, hip joints, and upper femora, AP

Hand, AP

Knee or elbow region, AP

This protocol is flexible and can be expanded if there is a relevant clinical abnormality or if a more complete survey is deemed necessary after inspection of the initial radiographs.

c) Systematic radiological evaluation is essential if a correct diagnosis is to be reached. In all skeletal dysplasias the epiphyseal, metaphyseal and diaphyseal findings in the tubular bones must be evaluated. In the sclerosing bone dysplasias a 'head-to-foot' approach is advised, attempts at diagnosis being postponed until the total radiographic changes have been assessed in:

  i) skull and facial bones;

  ii) spine;

  iii) chest and pelvis;

  iv) tubular bones and extremities.

d) It is self-evident that before diagnosing bone sclerosis the radiologist must ensure that the radiographs are not underpenetrated. This rule also applies to copies of original films, as in these the overall contrast can be increased by overexposure. Overpenetrated films should be used with circumspection, but they may be required for demonstration of the extent of cortical involvement or the "bone within a bone" appearance in osteopetrosis.

e) In a review of the neurosurgical implications of the craniotubular dysplasias, KIRKPATRICK et al. (1977) drew attention to the possibility of stenosis of the foramen magnum due to bone overgrowth and advised radiographic assessment of this region before surgery.

f) Thin-section tomography is of value in the assessment of bony encroachment upon the foramina of the cranial nerves prior to surgical decompression, and in the evaluation of the base of the skull. Computerised tomography (CT) has proved to be disappointing in this type of investigation but is of value in the demonstration of absence of internal hydrocephalus and the extent of calvarial thickening prior to craniotomy in patients with elevated intracranial pressure (see Chaps. 13 and 20).

Taxonomy

Abnormal bone density may be regional or widely distributed. It may be complete or partial and possibly associated with modelling deficiency in some areas and hypoplasia in others. Eventually, it may be feasible to make an objective analysis of skeletal characteristics such as size, shape, contour and configuration, and thereby identify specific dysplasias.

An approach to taxonomy known as 'pattern profile analysis' has been developed by POZNANSKI et al. (1972). This technique involves measuring the lengths of metacarpals and phalanges on radiographs and expressing the results graphically in terms of the mean and standard deviation for normal individuals (Fig. 3-1). Pattern profile analysis is of limited value in the diagnosis of bone dysplasias, but it has potential for syndrome delineation and recognition of heterogeneity. An immediate application would be in determining the relationship, if any, between frontometaphyseal dysplasia and osteodysplasty.

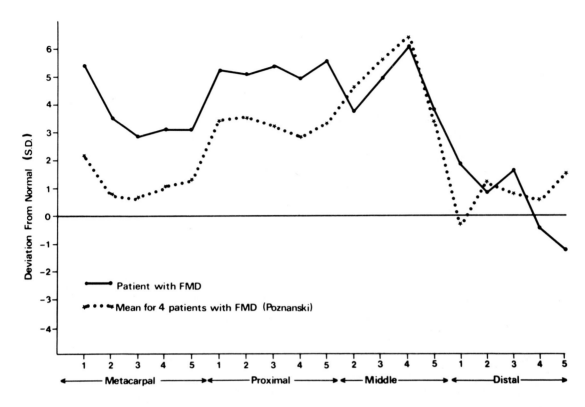

Fig. 3-1. Pattern profile analysis of the AP radiograph of the hand of an adult male with suspected frontometaphyseal dysplasia compared with the mean results from four known cases. The similarity of configuration of the two graphs supports the diagnosis. (The authors express their gratitude to Professor A.K. Poznanski, Michigan, U.S.A. for data contained in Fig. 3-1)

Terminology

Certain descriptive radiological terms are frequently employed in the context of the sclerosing bone dysplasias. They are sometimes erroneously interchanged but in fact they have specific connotations. For the sake of clarity, those which are the source of most confusion are defined below:

Sclerosis   Increase in density without any alteration in configuration.

Hyperostosis Increase in width and density of bone.

Modelling   Alteration of the contours and shape of a bone in normal growth and development.

Malformation A structural abnormality due to faulty development, e.g. the abnormal shape of the mandible in pycnodysostosis.

Deformity   An alteration in shape of a previously normal part, e.g. following a pathological fracture in osteopetrosis.

Dysplasia   Intrinsic faulty development of the whole skeleton.

Dysostosis   Malformation of individual bones, singly or in combination.

Some descriptive radiological terms of a nontechnical nature have proved to be of value. Examples are the 'policeman's nightstick or truncheon' configuration of the long bones in certain craniotubular hyperostoses and the 'Erlenmeyer flask' (Fig. 3-2a) expansion of the long bones, especially the distal femora, which is characteristic of Pyle disease. This latter appearance is also a feature, to a lesser extent, of some patients with osteopetrosis, craniometaphyseal dysplasia, frontometaphyseal dysplasia, osteodysplasty and the Schwarz-Lélek syndrome.

Differential Diagnosis

Conditions other than the sclerosing bone dysplasias in which the skeleton becomes dense are reviewed in Chap. 22. Distinguishing features of disorders where the femur has an Erlenmeyer flask configuration are as follows:

a) Thalassaemia (Fig. 3-2b). The calvarium shows thickening and spiculation, and the skeleton has a coarse trabecular pattern.

b) Gaucher disease (Fig. 3-2c). Patchy areas of sclerosis and lysis may be evident, particularly in the upper femur. The spleen is usually enlarged.

c) Lead poisoning. Transverse bands of increased bone density appear in the metaphyses. These changes resemble those of the infantile form of osteopetrosis.

The lower femora are expanded in diaphyseal achalasia and Ollier disease, but asymmetry and the presence of multiple exostoses or enchondromata respectively indicates the true diagnosis.

It is of passing interest that the classical Erlenmeyer flask configuration was evident in a radiograph of the left lower limb of a Nubian mummy (SMITH and JONES 1910). However, there were no other features to permit a firm diagnosis in this particular case!

References

KIRKPATRICK DB, RIMOIN DL, KAITILA I, GOODMAN SJ (1977) The craniotubular bone modelling disorders: A neurosurgical introduction to rare skeletal dysplasias with cranial nerve compression. Surg Neurol 7:221

POZNANSKI AK, GARN SM, NAGY JM, GALL JC (1972) Metacarpophalangeal pattern profiles in the evaluation of skeletal malformations. Radiology 104:1

SMITH GE, JONES FW (1910) The archaeological survey of Nubia. Report for 1907–1908, vol. 2, Cairo

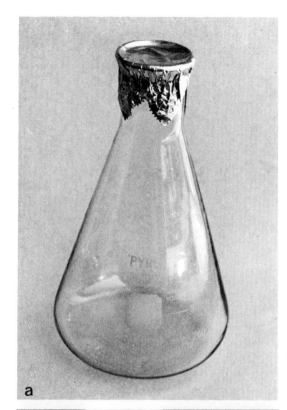

Fig. 3-2. (a) Erlenmeyer flask, a glass container widely used in chemical laboratories. (b) Thalassaemia. The distal portion of the femur has the Erlenmeyer flask configuration. (c) Gaucher disease. This disorder enters into the differential diagnosis of the Erlenmeyer flask appearance

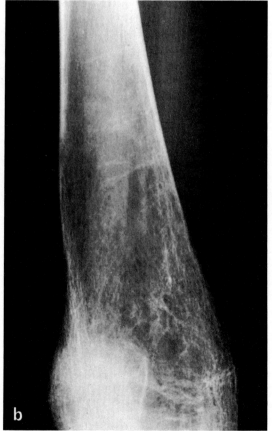

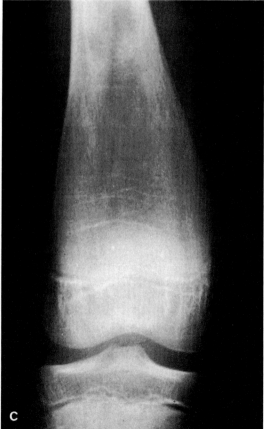

Chapter 4
Osteopetrosis

Historical and Nosological Considerations

The first clear-cut description of osteopetrosis is attributed to a German radiologist, ALBERS-SCHÖNBERG (1904), who reported a 26-year-old male with generalised skeletal sclerosis and multiple fractures. SCHULZE (1921) used the term 'marble bones' ('Marmorknochen') in conjunction with the eponym 'Albers-Schönberg,' and in a radiological review KARSHNER (1926) subsequently introduced the designation 'osteopetrosis.'

It became evident that the clinical course was very variable, and McPEAK (1936) proposed subdivision of osteopetrosis into 'malignant' and 'benign' types. RUBIN (1964) emphasised the early development of complications in the former variety by advocating the categories 'congenital' and 'tarda'. The alternative designations 'precocious' and 'delayed' have been preferred in the Paris Nomenclature, and it is generally accepted that the former variety is transmitted as an autosomal recessive, while the latter is an autosomal dominant.

The osteopetroses are categorised in the following way:

Osteopetrosis with precocious manifestations: congenital, malignant autosomal recessive form.

Osteopetrosis with delayed manifestations: tarda, benign, autosomal dominant form.

Although a large proportion of patients fall into one or other of these groups, there have been numerous atypical cases, and this classification certainly oversimplifies the true situation. It is probable that there is heterogeneity within each of these categories and that there are 'intermediate' forms which are clinically and genetically distinct.

Clinical Features

The benign form of osteopetrosis often remains clinically silent and is recognised only by chance or following family studies. Alternatively, facial palsy or deafness due to cranial nerve compression may draw attention to the underlying skeletal sclerosis. In some individuals the skeleton is fragile, and pathological fractures may occur. However, there is disagreement concerning the physical properties of the skeleton, and surgical colleagues have likened the texture of the bone at operation to both 'chalk' and 'cheese.' This observation may well be indicative of heterogeneity.

The malignant form of osteopetrosis is a serious condition which presents in infancy with dyshaemopoesis, hepatosplenomegaly, and failure to thrive. Cranial nerve palsies often develop and there is usually a fatal outcome in early childhood. Many patients have clinical problems which fall somewhere between these extremes and 'intermediate' cases are not uncommon. This situation is of practical importance in prognostication and genetic counselling.

A propensity to osteomyelitis, especially of the mandible, is a problem in some patients, and the successful management of this complication with hyperbaric oxygen represents an important therapeutic advance (MAINOUS et al. 1975). If bony encroachment develops, surgical decompression of the facial nerve is of proven value (HAMERSMA 1970, 1974). Degenerative osteoarthritis of the hip joint may be a primary phenomenon or occur as a consequence of coxa vara, and prosthetic joint replacement has been undertaken with good results (CAMERON and DEWAR 1977). The place of corticosteroids and bone marrow transplantation for haematological complications in the 'lethal' form of osteopetrosis is still a matter of controversy.

Radiographic Manifestations

Generalised symmetrical skeletal sclerosis is the hallmark of osteopetrosis. The changes are age-related and there is variation in severity and distribution between affected persons. The radiographic features have been reviewed by HINKEL and BEILER (1955), GRAHAM et al. (1973), and BEIGHTON et al. (1979).

Skull

In the young, sclerosis is more prominent at the base than in the vault, and in the anteroposterior view the dense orbits and sphenoid bones produce a classic 'mask' sign. Calvarial sclerosis develops, and although thickening is not pronounced the sinuses may not be visualised. In the 'malignant' form, encroachment upon the optic nerve foramina may begin at an early stage.

In the adult, sclerosis of the calvarium becomes more obvious, and although involvement of the mandible can reach a moderate degree, there is little or no facial distortion. Osteomyelitis of the jaw may occur in all forms of osteopetrosis.

Spine

In the young, 'endobones' are visible within the vertebral bodies. This striking feature of osteopetrosis may be demonstrated to the best advantage by penetrated views. The endobones represent the original dense bone which is present at birth. In the adult, sclerosis of the end plates gives a striped 'sandwich' or 'rugger jersey' appearance. The posterior elements of the vertebrae also show sclerotic changes, usually of mild degree.

Chest and Pelvis

In childhood, endobones may be present in the ribs and pelvis, while the iliac wings may contain convex arcs of sclerotic bone. These changes disappear by adulthood and the end result is a diffuse, ground-glass appearance. The external contours of these bones are undisturbed.

Limbs

The major feature in the bones of the limbs is sclerosis, with endobone formation, striations and modelling defects predominating in the young.

In infancy, diffuse sclerosis is present throughout the limbs. It is difficult to separate the cortex from the medulla and this feature distinguishes osteopetrosis from the much less severe physiological sclerosis of the newborn. The metaphyseal regions may show a terminal area of lucent irregularity and the increased fragility of these regions results in linear fractures. In the past, this appearance has erroneously been likened to rickets.

In childhood, endobone or 'os in os' formation is evident in the long and short tubular bones and the small bones of wrists and ankles. Prior to obliteration, endobones may appear to be displaced and lie eccentrically in the shafts of the tubular bones.

The modelling defects take the form of clubbing or flasking of the bone ends. These changes develop at the most rapidly growing regions and are seen particularly in the distal femur and proximal humerus. In these areas multiple transverse stratifications and longitudinal striations are evident; these represent differing degrees of bone formation and resorption.

In the adult some of the childhood features may persist, but as growth ceases, the scleroses become uniform and regular, producing dense bones with thickened cortices.

Bone fragility is inconsistent, but if fractures occur, they are typically transverse with sharp margins and situated in densely sclerotic areas. They usually heal rapidly and produce little deformity, but delayed union is occasionally a problem. Coxa vara may result from fracture and deformity of the femoral neck.

Comment

The terms 'osteopetrosis' or 'Albers-Schönberg disease' have often been used loosely in the past for a variety of craniotubular dysplasias and hyperostoses, and the early literature should be interpreted with caution. For instance, the reports by SEIGMAN and KILBY (1950) and PALMER and THOMAS (1958) pertain to patients with pycnodysostosis. The problem of semantics and differential diagnosis has been reviewed by BEIGHTON et al. (1977) and HORAN and BEIGHTON (1978).

Osteopetrosis, in the strict sense of the term, is fairly common and more than 500 cases have now been described. The majority have been of the benign autosomal dominant type, and JOHNSTON et al. (1968) were able to recognise this form of osteopetrosis in 19 kindreds, containing 85 affected persons. MONTGOMERY and STANDARD (1960) gave an account of variable clinical and radiographic features in a Jamaican kindred in which a mother and eight offspring were affected.

The malignant autosomal recessive form is distinctly rare; amongst the few clear reports are those of ENELL and PEHRSON (1958), TIPS and LYNCH (1962) and KOZLOWSKI et al. (1972). The abnormal gene evidently reaches a high frequency in Costa Rica: LORIA-CORTES et al. (1977) encountered 26 affected boys and girls in 12 families. Survival into adulthood has been recorded in 'malignant' osteopetrosis (DICK and SIMPSON 1972), and it appears that the initial clinical manifestations are not always indicative of the eventual outcome.

Apart from the problem of multiple designations for osteopetrosis, the term 'tarda' is certainly a misnomer. Indeed, DELAHAYE et al. (1976) made a fortuitous diagnosis of this type of osteopetrosis in a mother and her unborn child during radiopelvimetry. There is undoubtedly considerable heterogeneity and there are many examples of anomalous inheritance and atypical clinical and radiographic features. Precise delineation will probably have to await elucidation of the basic defect.

References

ALBERS-SCHÖNBERG H (1904) Röntgenbilder einer seltenen Knochenerkrankung. Münch Med Wochenschr 51:365

BEIGHTON P, HORAN FT, HAMERSMA H (1977) A review of the osteopetroses. Postgrad Med J 53:507

BEIGHTON P, HAMERSMA H, CREMIN BJ (1979) Osteopetrosis in South Africa. The benign, lethal and intermediate forms. S Afr Med J 55:659

CAMERON HU, DEWAR FP (1977) Degenerative osteoarthritis associated with osteopetrosis. Clin Orthop 127:148

DELAHAYE RP, METGES PJ, ANGLADE JP, MALMEZAT X, PASCAL-SUISSE P (1976) Découverte simultanée d'une ostéopétrose chez la mère et le foetus à l'occasion d'une radiopelvimétrie. J Radiol Electrol Med Nucl 57:359

DICK HM, SIMPSON WJ (1972) Dental changes in osteopetrosis. Oral Surg 34:408

ENELL H, PEHRSON M (1958) Studies on osteopetrosis. 1. Clinical report of three cases with genetic considerations. Acta Paediatr 47:279

GRAHAM CB, RUDHE U, EKLÖF O (1973) Osteopetrosis. In: Kaufmann HJ (ed.) Intrinsic diseases of bones. Karger, Basel (Progress in pediatric radiology, vol 4, p 375)

HAMERSMA H (1970) Osteopetrosis (marble bone disease) of the temporal bone. Laryngoscope 80 10:1518

HAMERSMA H (1974) Total decompression of the facial nerve in osteopetrosis (marble bone disease – morbus Albers-Schönberg). J Otolaryngol 36:21

HINKEL CL, BEILER DD (1955) Osteopetrosis in adults. A J R 74:46

HORAN FT, BEIGHTON P (1978) Osteopetrosis in the Fairbank collection. J Bone Joint Surg [Br] 60:53

JOHNSTON CC, LAVY N, LORD T, VELLIOS F. MERRITT AD, DEISS WP (1968) Osteopetrosis. A clinical, genetic, metabolic and morphologic study of the dominantly inherited, benign form. Medicine (Baltimore) 47:149

KARSHNER RG (1926) Osteopetrosis. A J R 16:405

KOZLOWSKI K, SZMIGIEL C, KONIK R. OSTROWSKI A, WALECKI J (1972) Osteopetrosis with precocious manifestations. Australas Radiol 16:311

LORIA-CORTES R, QUESADA-CALVO E. CORDERO-CHAVERRI C (1977) Osteopetrosis in children: A report of 26 cases. J Pediatr 91:43

MAINOUS EG, HART GB, SOFFA DJ, GRAHAM GA (1975) Hyperbaric oxygen treatment of mandibular Osteomyelitis in osteopetrosis. J Oral Surg 33:288

MCPEAK CN (1936) osteopetrosis: Report of eight cases occurring in three generations of one family. A J R 36:816

MONTGOMERY RD, STANDARD KL (1960) Albers-Schönberg's disease: A changing concept. J Bone Joint Surg [Br] 42:303

PALMER PES, THOMAS JEP (1958) Osteopetrosis with unusual changes in the skull and digits. Br J Radiol 31:705

RUBIN P (1964) Dynamic classification of bone dysplasias. Year Book Medical Publishers, Chicago, p 258

SCHULZE F (1921) Das Wesen des Krankheitsbildes der 'Marmorknochen' (Albers-Schönberg). Arch Klin Chir 118:411

SEIGMAN EL, KILBY WL (1950) Osteopetrosis. Report of a case and review of recent literature. A J R 63:865

TIPS RL, LYNCH HT (1962) Malignant congenital osteopetrosis resulting from a consanguineous marriage. Acta Paediatr 51:585

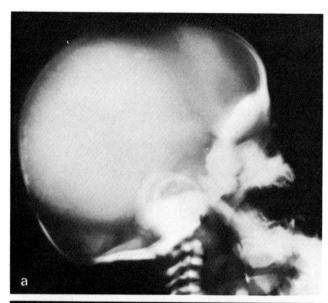

Osteopetrosis is depicted in an infant, a child and an adult. Case 1 is presented by kind permission of Dr. John Masel, Brisbane, Australia. Cases 4, 5, and 6 are included in order to demonstrate the spectrum of changes in affected adults

Case I
Two-month-old infant

Fig. 4-1. (a) Skull. Sclerosis is evident in the calvarium, base and frontal bones

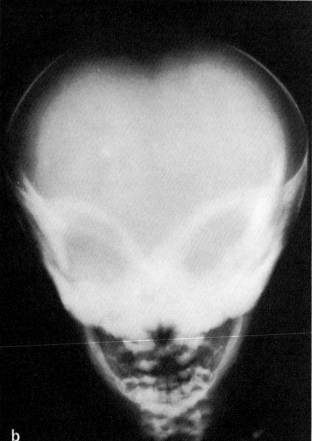

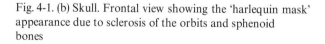

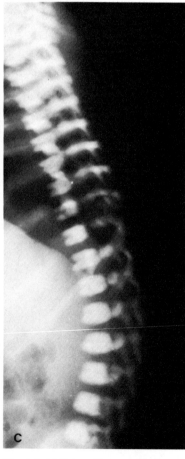

Fig. 4-1. (b) Skull. Frontal view showing the 'harlequin mask' appearance due to sclerosis of the orbits and sphenoid bones

Fig. 4-1. (c) Spine. The vertebral bodies and their appendages are dense. The anterior lucent notches are produced by vascular channels

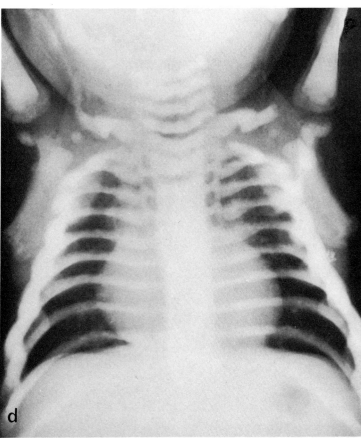

Fig. 4-1. (d) Chest. All bones are uniformly dense. Growth disturbance is present at the inferior margins of the scapulae and periosteal reaction is evident around the proximal humeri

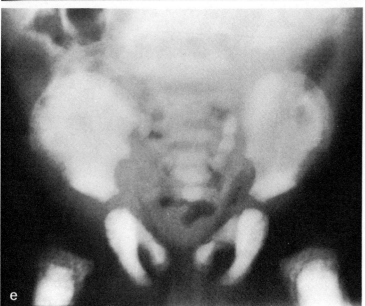

Fig. 4-1. (e) Pelvis. Generalised sclerosis and growth disturbance are noted in the iliac wings and proximal femora

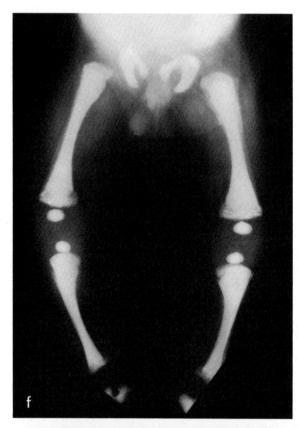

Fig. 4-1. (f and g) Limbs. These are uniformly dense and there is a frayed 'pseudorickets' appearance at the growing metaphyses. These areas are abnormally fragile and fractures have occurred. (h) Enlarged view of the forearm to demonstrate fractures through the metaphyses of the distal ulna and radius, with periosteal reaction

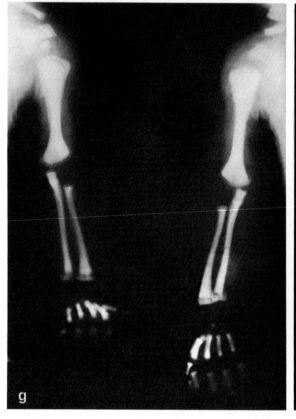

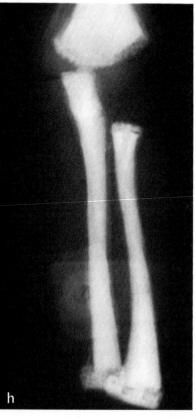

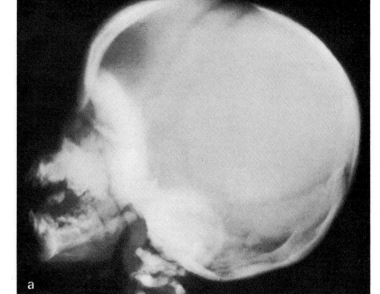

Case II
Boy aged 1 year (Beighton et al. 1979)

Fig. 4-2. (a) Skull. Increased thickening and density are present in the vault, base and maxilla

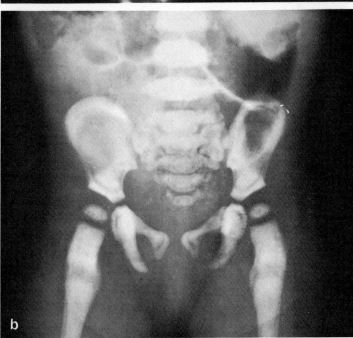

Fig. 4-2. (b) Pelvis. The pelvis and proximal femora show bands of sclerosis in the growing bones. A 'bone within a bone' appearance is seen in the iliac wings and lack of modelling and vertical striations are evident in the femoral metaphyses

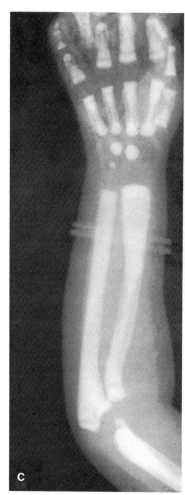

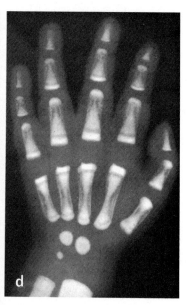

Fig. 4-2. (c) Arm. Sclerosis of the arm bones with undermodelling of the distal radius and upper humerus. (d) Hand. Endobones are present in the metacarpals and phalanges. It is of interest that in the phalanges the endobones are broad at their epiphyseal bases, whilst in the matacarpals they are wide at both ends

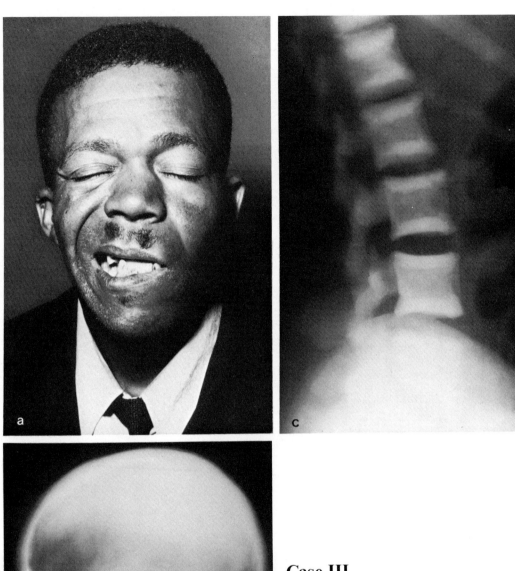

Case III
Male aged 40 years (Beighton et al. 1979)

Fig. 4-3. (a) Apart from left-sided palsy, the patient is clinically normal. (b) Skull. The base, calvarium and maxilla are sclerotic and the air spaces are unpneumatised. (c) Spine. Sclerosis of vertebral bodies, which is marked at the superior and inferior surfaces, produces the classical 'rugger jersey' appearance (Beighton et al. 1977)

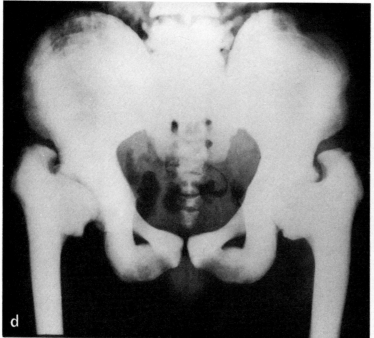

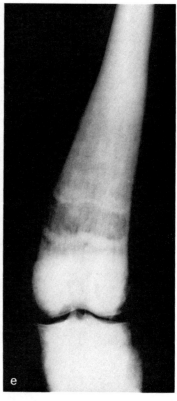

Fig. 4-3. (d) Pelvis. All bones show diffuse density and deformities are present in the femoral necks. (e) Distal femur with lack of modelling, dense sclerosis and transverse and vertical lines of increased density

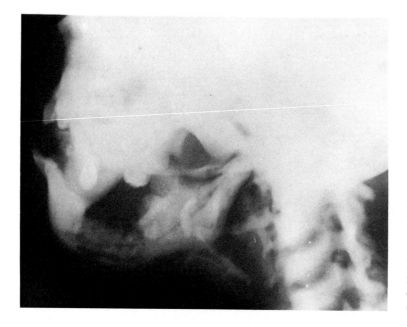

Case IV
Female aged 22

Fig. 4-4. Oblique view of the mandible showing areas of destruction due to osteomyelitis (Beighton et al. 1979)

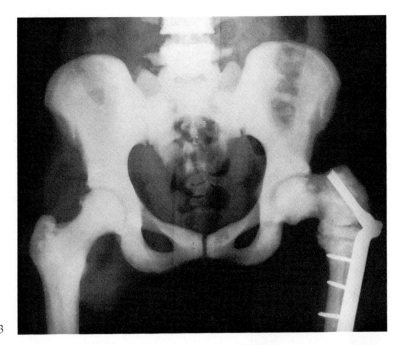

Case V
Female aged 33

Fig. 4-5. Pelvis, showing well-marked sclerosis and a pathological fracture in the left hip

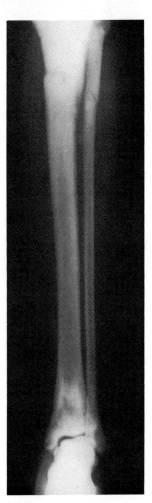

Case VI
Male aged 31

Fig. 4-6. Typical transverse pathological fractures are present in the upper tibia and fibula

Chapter 5

Pycnodysostosis

Historical and Nosological Considerations

Pycnodysostosis was delineated by MAROTEAUX and LAMY (1962), the designation being derived from the Greek 'pycnos' and having the connotation 'dense bones'.

Prior to this definitive description, the condition had been confused with osteopetrosis, due to the generalised skeletal density, and with cleidocranial dysostosis, on the basis of clavicular hypoplasia and persistence of the fontanelles. The earliest recognisable case was reported by MONTANARI (1923) and more than 100 patients in 50 kindreds have now been described.

There have been many instances of parental consanguinity or affected siblings with normal parents, and autosomal recessive inheritance is well established. The clinical and genetic features have been reviewed by ELMORE (1967) and SEDANO et al. (1968).

Clinical Features

Short stature is a major feature of pycnodysostosis and adult height ranges between 130 and 150 cm.

The terminal phalanges are short and splayed, with hypoplasia of the nails; genu valgus and pectus excavatum are variable features.

The head is relatively large with frontal and occipital prominence, the nose is pointed and hooked, and the chin recedes. Characteristically, the angle of the mandible is obtuse, while the eyes may be exophthalmic with some blueing of the sclerae. The palate is high, and dental malocclusion and caries are common. Affected individuals, even of different ethnic groups, have a strong facial resemblance to one another.

General health is good, but the skeleton is fragile and multiple fractures may occur.

Radiographic Manifestations

Generalised skeletal sclerosis without significant disturbance of modelling is the main abnormality. This sclerosis may be of minor degree in infancy but increases progressively during growth. The radiographic features of pycnodysostosis have been reviewed by MAROTEAUX and FAURÉ (1973).

Skull

In the skull the calvarium and base are sclerotic, the orbital rims are dense, and the mastoid air sinuses are obliterated. The fontanelles and sutures, especially the lambdoid, are wide during early childhood and this feature may lead to a misdiagnosis of hydrocephalus. The fontanelles remain patent in adulthood and Wormian bones are usually evident in the parietal sutures. Micrognathia and an obtuse mandibular angle are consistent manifestations. The facial bones are hypoplastic and the paranasal sinuses are small.

Spine

The vertebral bodies are sclerotic but their transverse processes are spared. In the adult the bodies may be spool-shaped, due to anterior and posterior concavities. The neural arches may remain unfused, and spondylolisthesis in the lumbosacral region is not uncommon.

Chest and Pelvis

The ribs are uniformly dense and the clavicles show variable hypoplasia of their lateral portions. In the pelvis the acetabula are shallow and angulated, and coxa valgus or varus may be present.

Limbs

The long bones have dense cortices, narrow medullary cavities, and undisturbed external contours. Massive callus formation and the sequelae of multiple pathological fractures may be evident. The tibiae are sometimes bowed and the bones of the forearm may show a Madelung deformity.
The distal portions of the terminal phalanges become increasingly dysplastic throughout infancy and may eventually resemble acro-osteolysis. This fragmentation is not uniform and the occasional bone may be spared. The adjacent phalanges take on a frayed or pointed appearance and the other tubular bones of the hands and feet may be somewhat short.

Comment

Maroteaux and Lamy (1965) suggested that the impressionist painter Toulouse-Lautrec might have had pycnodysostosis. His short stature, facial appearance, and bone fragility are certainly in accordance with this theory. Although pycnodysostosis is relatively uncommon, it has a wide geographical distribution. Besides Western Europe and North America, cases have been reported from India (Diwan and Gogate 1974), Israel (Roth 1976) and Indonesia (Srivastava et al. 1978). The condition seems to be particularly common in Japan; 29 cases have been reported by Sugiura et al. (1974) and Kawahara et al. (1977). In our own experience we have encountered pycnodysostosis in patients of Negro stock from Rhodesia, Malawi and South Africa.

There have been several reports of atypical forms of pycnodysostosis. For instance, Kozlowski and Yu (1972) described an Australian child with the additional features of hepatosplenomegaly, anaemia and rickets. Similarly, in craniomandibular dermatodysostosis, dermal lesions are associated with patchy lysis and sclerosis of the long bones, clavicular hypoplasia, acro-osteolysis, micrognathia, Wormian bones and delayed closure of the fontanelles. Danks et al. (1974) reported a six-year-old boy with this disorder and pointed out that although some features were reminiscent of pycnodysostosis, it was clearly a separate entity.

The unique cranial and digital abnormalities facilitate recognition of pycnodysostosis, and the radiological differentiation from osteopetrosis and cleidocranial dysplasia is an easy matter. Distinguishing features are given in Table 5-1.

Table 5-1. Distinguishing features of pycnodysostosis, osteopetrosis and cleidocranial dysplasia

	Pycnodysostosis	Osteopetrosis	Cleidocranial dysplasia
Skeletal sclerosis	Uniform	Modelling defects and striations	Nil
Skull: Patent sutures	+	Nil	+
Wormian bones	+	Nil	+
Angle of jaw	Very obtuse	Nil	Mildly obtuse
Terminal phalanges	Absorption	Nil	Nil
Clavicular hypoplasia	Mild	Nil	+
Dental anomalies	+	Sometimes	Nil
Bone fragility	+	Sometimes	Nil

References

DANKS DM, MAYNE V, NORMAN H, WETTENHALL B, HALL RK (1974) Craniomandibular dermatodysostosis. Birth Defects 10 12:99

DIWAN RV, GOGATE AN (1974) Pycnodysostosis (first report of a family from India). Indian J Radiol 28:268

ELMORE SM (1967) Pycnodysostosis: A review. J Bone Joint Surg [Am] 49:153

KAWAHARA K, NISHIKIORI M, IMAI K, KSIHI K, FUJIKI Y (1977) Radiographic observations of pyknodysostosis: Report of a case. Oral Surg 44/3:476

KOZLOWSKI K, YU JS (1972) Pycnodysostosis. A variant form with visceral manifestations. Arch Dis Child 47:804

MAROTEAUX P, FAURÉ C (1973) Pycnodysostosis. Prog Pediatr Radiol 4:403

MAROTEAUX P, LAMY M (1962) La pycnodysostose. Presse Méd 70:999

MAROTEAUX P, LAMY M (1965) The malady of Toulouse-Lautrec. J A M A 191:111

MONTANARI U (1923) Acondroplasia e disostosi cleidocrania digitale. Arch Putti Chir Organi Mov 7:379

ROTH VG (1976) Pycnodysostosis presenting with bilateral subtrochanteric fractures: Case report. Clin Orthop 117:247

SEDANO HD, GORLIN RJ, ANDERSON VE (1968) Pycnodysostosis. Clinical and genetic considerations. Am J Dis Child 116:70

SRIVASTAVA KK, BHATTACHARYA AK, GALATIUS-JENSEN F, TAMAELA LA, BORGSTEIN A, KOZLOWSKI K (1978) Pycnodysostosis (Report of four cases). Australas Radiol 22:70

SUGIURA Y, AMADO Y, KOH J (1974) Pycnodysostosis in Japan. Report of six cases and a review of Japanese literature. Birth Defects 10:78

Two cases are shown to illustrate the age-related appearances in infancy and adulthood. The first patient, at 6 months of age, provides the earliest recorded radiographic description of pycnodysostosis

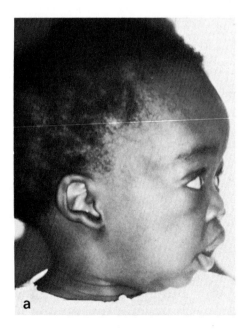

Case I
Infant, aged 6 months

Fig. 5-1. (a) The forehead is bossed and the chin recedes

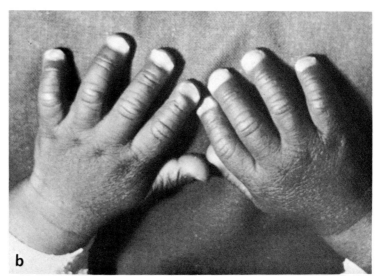

Fig. 5-1. (b) The hands are stubby, with short terminal phalanges

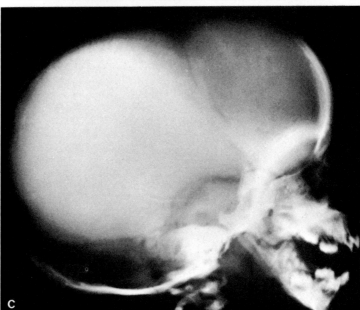

Fig. 5-1. (c) Skull. Sclerosis of the parietal bone, splayed sutures and an open anterior fontanelle are present. The facial bones are relatively hypoplastic and the mandibular angle is wide

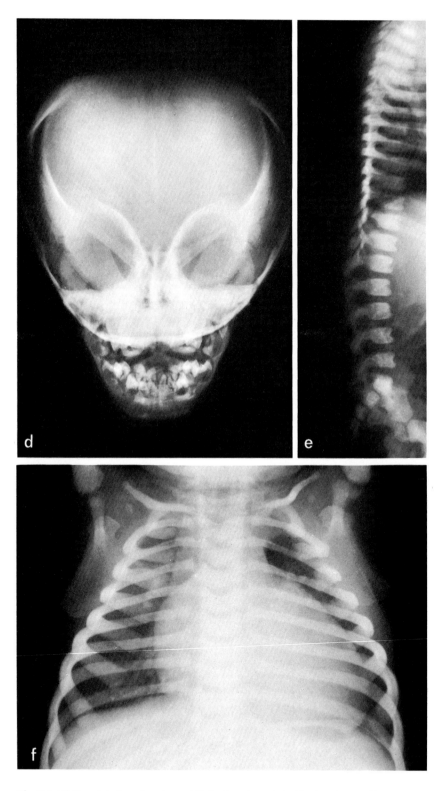

Fig. 5-1. (d) Frontal view showing orbital sclerosis and the 'harlequin mask' appearance, which resembles that of osteopetrosis. (e) Spine. Sclerosis is not marked in early infancy. (f) Chest. Hypoplasia of the acromial ends of the clavicles is a variable feature and was not present in any of our patients

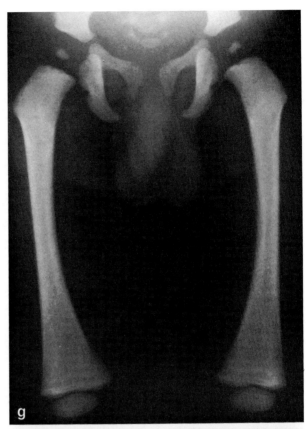

Fig. 5-1. (g) Femora. At this stage the long
bones are relatively normal

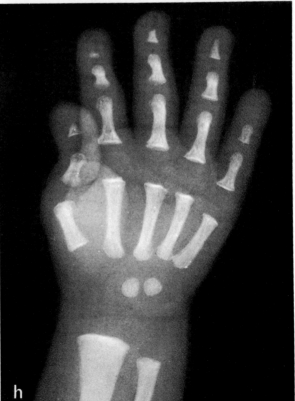

Fig. 5-1. (h) Hand showing asymmetrical
hypoplasia of the terminal phalanges. The
terminal phalanx of the 5th digit is not visible

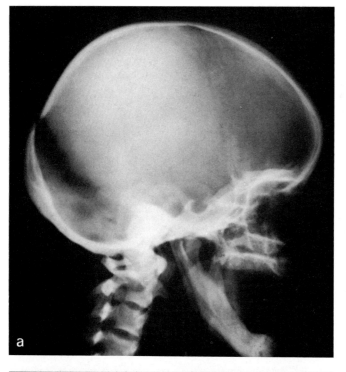

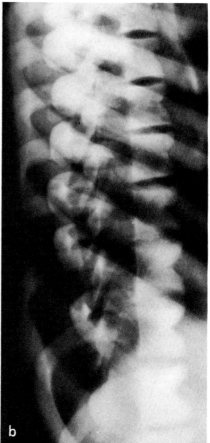

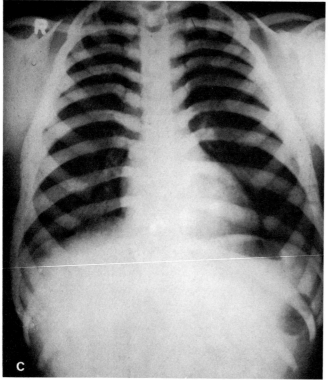

Case II
Male aged 30 years

Fig. 5-2. (a) Skull. Sclerosis is most marked in the parietal bones. The lamboid sutures have remained open, the facial bones are small and the sinuses are poorly aerated. The mandible has a markedly obtuse angle and is edentulous. (b) Spine. The vertebral bodies have a 'spool' appearance due to anterior concavities. (c) Chest. Diffuse sclerosis is evident. The clavicles are normal

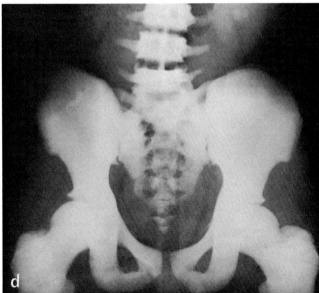

Fig. 5-2. (d) Pelvis. The pelvis and proximal femora are sclerotic but their external contours are undisturbed

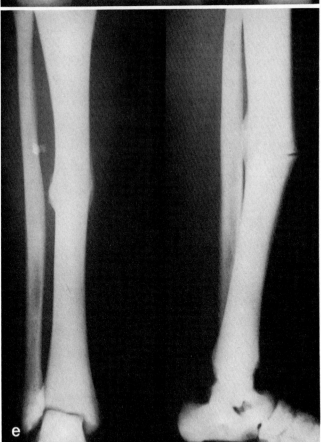

Fig. 5-2. (e) Limbs. The bones are diffusely sclerotic and the tibiae show transverse fractures with callus formation

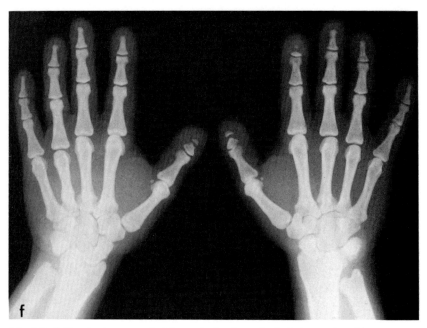

Fig. 5-2. (f) Hands. Asymmetrical hypoplasia of terminal phalanges is evident

Chapter 6

Metaphyseal Dysplasia
(Pyle Disease)

Historical and Nosological Considerations

Under the title 'A case of unusual bone development,' a Connecticut orthopaedic surgeon, EDWIN PYLE (1931), reported a healthy 5-year-old boy in
whom the mild clinical feature of knock-knees contrasted with gross undermodelling of the metaphyses of the tubular bones. BAKWIN and KRIDA
(1937) restudied this patient, together with his affected younger sister, and
termed the condition 'familial metaphyseal dysplasia.' Subsequently, HER-
MEL et al. (1953), KOMINS (1954), and FELD et al. (1954) employed the same
designation in descriptions of pairs of affected siblings who presented in
adulthood.

JACKSON et al. (1954) delineated craniometaphyseal dysplasia, a disorder
characterised by sclerosis of the cranium and defective modelling of the
metaphyses (see Chap. 7). The distinction between this condition and Pyle
disease was not widely appreciated, and a number of authors used the term
'Pyle disease' in reports of patients who clearly had craniometaphyseal dysplasia. Considerable semantic confusion ensued, but the situation was clari-
fied when GORLIN et al. (1969, 1970) emphasised the differences between
these separate entities.

The designation 'metaphyseal dysplasia (Pyle)' was employed in the 1970
and 1977 versions of the Paris Nomenclature, but in deference to popular
usage the eponymous form is retained in the text of this chapter.

About 20 genuine examples of Pyle disease are recognisable in the literature
and are listed in Table 6-1.

Clinical Features

Pyle disease is a benign condition, and general health and life span are
unimpaired. The only consistent external manifestations are genu valgus,
mild limitation of extension of the elbows, and palpable widening of the
clavicles. The teeth may be carious or misplaced, and a minority of affected
individuals have some degree of bone fragility, spinal malalignment or
prognathism. Several reported patients have been of tall stature, with dis-
proportionate lengthening of their limbs. Cranial nerve compression and
dyshaemopoesis do not occur.

Table 6-1. Published reports of Pyle disease

Authors	Patients	Country of origin
PYLE (1931)	Male aged 5	U.S.A.
COHN (1933)	Male	Germany
BAKWIN and KRIDA (1937)	Pyle's patient and sister aged 8	U.S.A. (Irish-American)
HERMEL et al. (1953)	Brother and sister aged 33 and 34	U.S.A.
FELD et al. (1954)	Brother and sister aged 53 and 46	U.S.A.
REVIGLIO (1954)	Female	Germany
KOMINS (1954)	Brother and sister aged 18 and 38	South Africa (English)
FORESTIER and GUILLEMINOT (1956)	Male	France
DANIEL (1960)	2 brothers	India
GORLIN et al. (1970)	Brothers aged 47 and 49	U.S.A.
TOGNOLO and MANARESI (1964)	Brother and sister	Italy
MABILLE et al. (1973)	Female aged 54[a]	France
RAAD and BEIGHTON (1978)	Male and female aged 20 and 24, distantly related[a]	South Africa (Afrikaner)

[a] Parental consanguinity.

Radiographic Manifestations

Gross undermodelling of the metaphyses of the tubular bones in association with mild cranial sclerosis are the significant radiographic features. These changes and their differential diagnosis have been reviewed by GORLIN et al. (1970), MABILLE et al. (1973) and HESELSON et al. (1979).

Skull

Involvement of the skull is limited to mild sclerosis of the calvarium and more density of the base. Enlargement of the brow and mandible are minor, variable features.

Spine

Changes in the spine are not remarkable, but minimal platyspondyly may be evident.

Chest and Pelvis

The medial portions of the clavicles are noticeably widened, with thinning of their cortices, and the sternal ends of the ribs show a lesser degree of expansion. In the pelvis, the pubic and ischial bones are also expanded.

Limbs

The metaphyses of the long bones show massive expansion, which extends into the shafts. The cortices are thin and these areas present an overall radiolucent appearance. These changes are most marked in the femur, where the configuration of the lower part has been likened to that of an Erlenmeyer flask. The proximal portion of the humerus and distal regions of the radius and ulna are also expanded, and similar changes are evident in the proximal regions of the tibia and fibula. In the bones of the lower limbs the mid-diaphyseal regions may show endosteal cortical thickening and the tibial shafts are sometimes slightly bowed.

Mild undermodelling is also present in the tubular bones of the extremities, with widening of the distal portions of the metacarpals and proximal regions of the phalanges.

Comment

From the practical point of view, the importance of Pyle disease lies in the awareness of the semantic confusion with craniometaphyseal dysplasia and in differentiation from other conditions which also manifest an Erlenmeyer flask deformity of the femur (see Chap. 3).

Several sets of affected siblings have been reported, and in some instances the parents have been consanguineous. Inheritance is autosomal recessive, and it is possible that the clinically asymptomatic heterozygous carrier of the gene can be detected by recognition of minor disturbances of modelling of the long bones (RAAD and BEIGHTON 1978).

Pyle disease is probably progressive throughout the period of growth, and the inconsistency of skull involvement in various reported cases may reflect the relative ages of the patients in question. Although PYLE (1931) did not mention radiographic changes in the skull of his first patient, SILVERMANN (1978) studied this individual again in later life and confirmed that the calvarium and base were sclerotic and oronasal sinuses and mastoids were poorly developed.

References

BAKWIN H, KRIDA A (1937) Familial metaphyseal dysplasia. Am J Dis Child 53:1521

BÜRGEL E, OLECK HG (1961) Familiäre metaphysäre Dysplasie. Fortschr Roentgenstr 94:460

COHN M (1933) Konstitutionelle Hyperspongiosierung des Skeletts mit partiellem Riesenwuchs. Fortschr Roentgenstr 47:293

DANIEL A (1960) Pyle's disease. Indian J Radiol 14:126

FELD H, SWITZER RA, DEXTER MW, LANGER EM (1954) Familial metaphyseal dysplasia. Radiology 65:206.

FORESTIER J, GUILLEMINOT R (1956) La maladie de Camurati-Engelmann. Rev Rhum Mal
    Ostéoartic 23:222
GORLIN RJ, SPRANGER J, KOSZALKA MF (1969) Genetic craniotubular bone dysplasias and
    hyperostoses; a critical analysis. Birth Defects 5/4:79
GORLIN RJ, KOSZALKA MF, SPRANGER J (1970) Pyle's disease (familial metaphyseal dys-
    plasia). J Bone Joint Surg [Am] 52:347
HERMEL MB, GERSHON-COHEN J, JONES DT (1953) Familial metaphyseal dysplasia. A J R
    70:413
HESELSON NG, RAAD MS, HAMERSMA H, CREMIN B, BEIGHTON P (1979) The radiological
    manifestations of metaphyseal dysplasia (Pyle disease). Br J Radiol 52:431
JACKSON WPU, ALBRIGHT F, DREWRY G, HANELIN J, RUBIN MI (1954) Metaphyseal dys-
    plasia, epiphyseal dysplasia, diaphyseal dysplasia and related conditions. Arch Intern
    Med 94/6:871
KOMINS C (1954) Familial metaphyseal dysplasia (Pyle's disease) Br J Radiol 27:670
MABILLE J-P, BENOIT J-P, CASTERA D (1973) Dysplasie métaphysaire de Pyle. Ann Radiol
    (Paris) 16/11:273
PYLE E (1931) A case of unusual bone development. J Bone Joint Surg 13:874
RAAD M, BEIGHTON P (1978) Autosomal recessive inheritance of metaphyseal dysplasia (Py-
    le disease). Clin Genet 14:251
REVIGLIO GM (1954) Rara osteopatia da turbe dell' accrescimento osseo. Malattia di Pyle.
    Minerva Med 1:418
TOGNOLO P, MANARESI C (1964) La displasia metafisaria famigliare. Arch Putti Chir Organi
    Mov 19:58

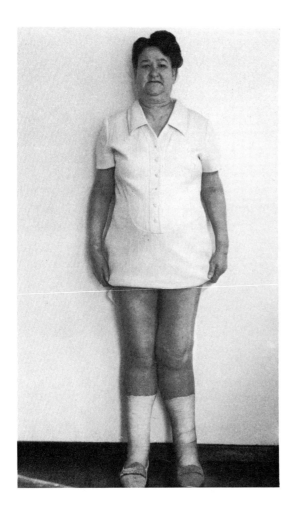

The radiographic features of three adults with Pyle disease are depicted. Patient 1, a female aged 24 years, and Patient 2, a male aged 20 years, are members of a consanguineous Afrikaner kindred and their pedigree is shown in Chap. 2. Patient 3 is an unrelated 45-year-old male. Figs. 6-2 to 6-7, 6-9 (b), 6-10, 6-11 (b) and 6-12 are from Heselson et al. 1979

Fig. 6-1. Patient 1. The face and habitus are normal except for genu valgum and widening of the transverse diameter of the knees (Raad and Beighton 1978)

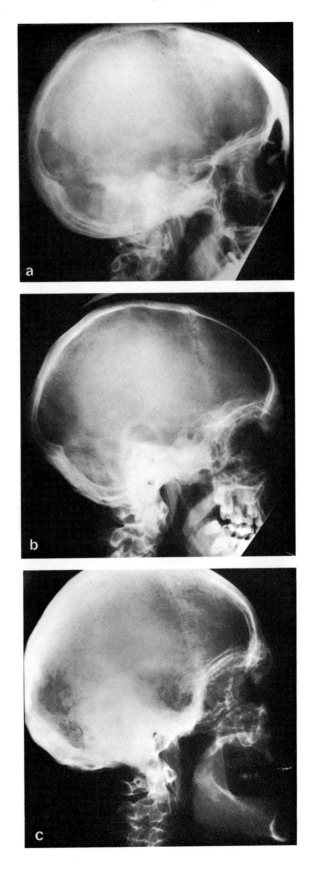

Fig. 6-2 a–c. Skull (a) Patient 1; (b) Patient 2; (c) Patient 3. In each patient the calvarium and base show patchy sclerosis and poor pneumatisation of the mastoid air cells and paranasal sinuses. Patient 3 has a distinct supra-orbital bulge, mild prognathism, and widening of the mandible

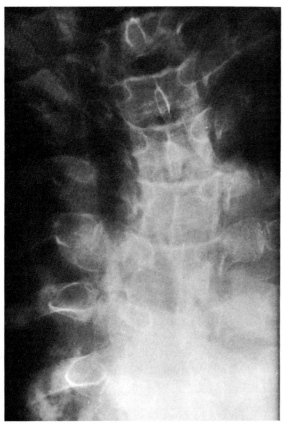

Fig. 6-3. Spine. Patient 1. Mild dorsal platyspondyly and scoliosis

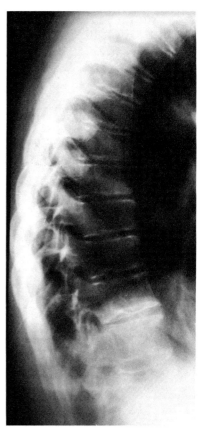

Fig. 6-4. Spine. Patient 3. Dorsal platyspondyly of mild degree

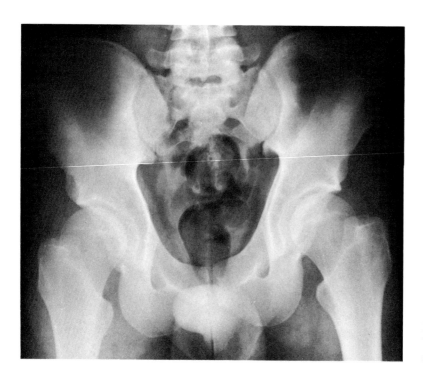

Fig. 6-5. Pelvis. Patient 2. Widening of the ischiopubic rami

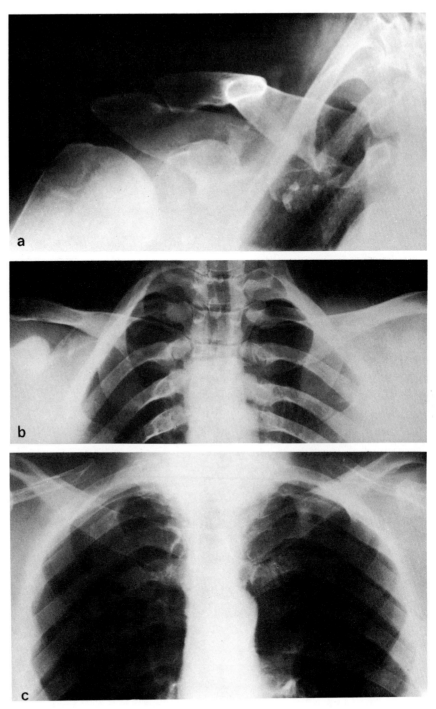

Fig. 6-6a–c. Thorax. (a) Patient 1; (b) Patient 2; (c) Patient 3. The clavicles show marked medial flaring. The ribs are widened to a lesser degree

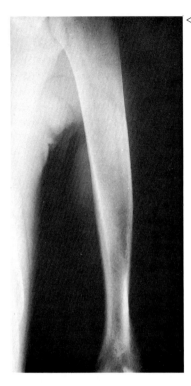

◁ Fig. 6-7. Arm. Patient 1. Undertubulation of the humerus in the proximal two-thirds

Fig. 6-8 a–c. Forearm. (a) Patient 1; (b) Patient 2; (c) Patient 3. Undertubulation of radius and ulna in their distal two-thirds
▽

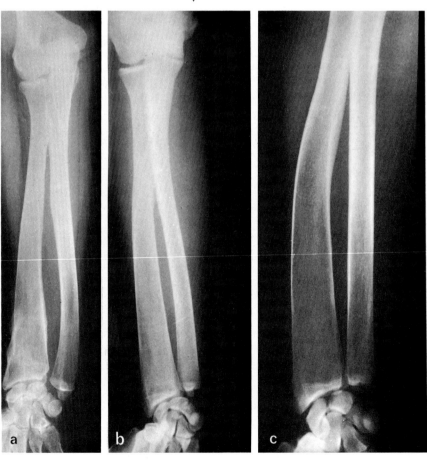

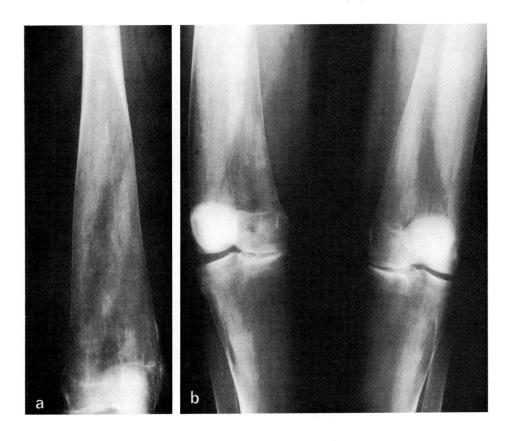

Fig. 6-9 a and b. Distal femur. (a) Patient 1;
(b) Patient 2. The femora exhibit gross Erlenmeyer
flask deformities and marked cortical thinning

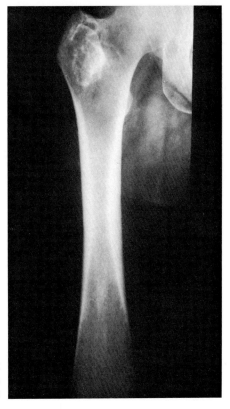

Fig. 6-10. Femur. Patient 1. The modelling defect
involves the mid-shaft and metaphyses and there is
endosteal cortical thickening of the mid-diaphysis

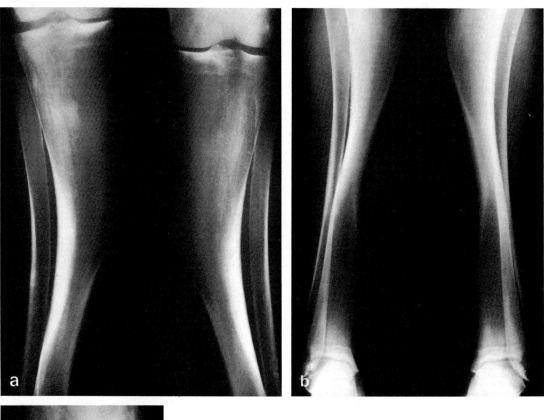

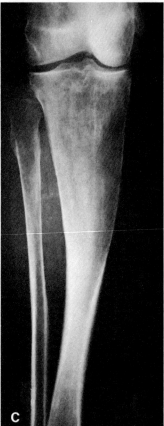

Fig. 6-11 a–c. Legs. (a) Patient 1; (b) Patient 2; (c) Patient 3. The tibiae show proximal flaring, undermodelling, and lateral S-shaped

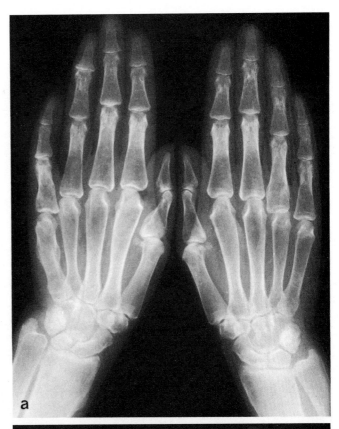

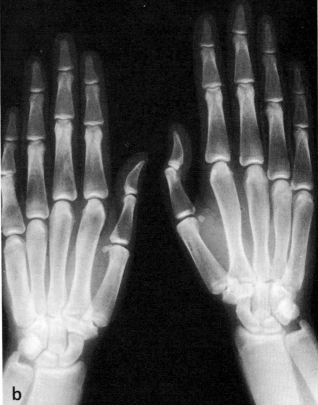

Fig. 6-12 a and b. Hands. (a) Patient 1;
(b) Patient 2. The metacarpals are
undermodelled distally and the phalanges
are wide proximally. Patient 1 has old
healed fractures of the right wrist and fifth
metacarpal

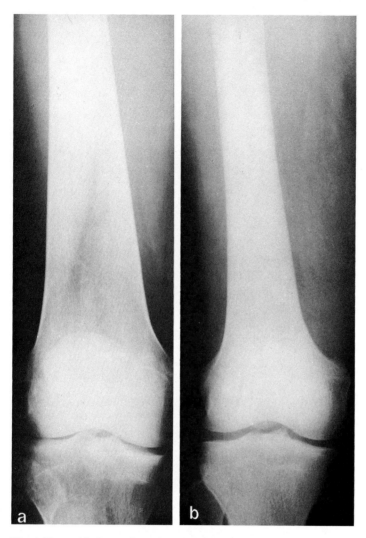

Fig. 6-13 a and b. Lower femora. (a) Mother of Patient 1; (b) Normal
40-year-old female. The distal femur in the mother of Patient 1,
a heterozygote or clinically normal carrier of the gene, shows mild
undertubulation compared with the normal female (Raad and Beighton
1978)

Chapter 7

Craniometaphyseal Dysplasia

Historical and Nosological Considerations

In a review of disorders of bone remodelling, JACKSON et al. (1954) expressed their belief that metaphyseal dysplasia could coexist with leontiasis ossea and sclerosis of the base of the skull in a distinct syndrome, which they designated 'craniometaphyseal dysplasia' (CMD). They identified five cases in the literature, three of which had been termed 'osteopetrosis' and two 'leontiasis ossea,' and added two patients of their own.

Once the syndromic status of CMD had been established, other reports followed. MORI and HOLT (1956) described three patients, one of whom had three affected relatives, and a similar dominant pattern of inheritance with generation-to-generation transmission was subsequently mentioned by several authors, including SPRANGER et al. (1965). Others reported kindreds in which transmission was apparently autosomal recessive (LEHMANN 1957; LIEVRE and FISCHGOLD 1956; MILLARD et al. 1967; ROSS and ALTMAN 1967), and it became evident that CMD was genetically heterogeneous.

GORLIN et al. (1969) pointed out that the clinical and radiographic features were much more severe in the recessive form than in the dominant type, and retrospectively several sporadic cases, including the two males in the original report of JACKSON et al. (1954), can be confidently assigned to the former category. It is now apparent that the autosomal dominant form is relatively common and the autosomal recessive type is rare.

Recent reports of CMD, which have been concerned with cranial nerve compression and in which autosomal dominant inheritance has been evident, have emanated from STOOL and CARUSO (1973), GARCIN et al. (1975), and MARTIN (1977).

Semantic confusion has persisted and several case reports concerning CMD have borne the title 'Pyle disease.' It must be emphasised that Pyle disease, described in Chap. 6, is separate and distinct from the dominant and recessive forms of CMD.

Clinical Features

The autosomal dominant type of CMD is a relatively benign disorder. Overgrowth of the skull may lead to mandibular prognathism as well as asymmetry, irregularity of the teeth and prominence of the forehead, but these changes are variable in degree and often relatively mild. Paranasal bossing is very obvious in infancy but becomes less marked in later life. Recurrent transient facial palsy occurs during childhood due to entrapment of the seventh cranial nerve, and the paralysis is sometimes permanent in adulthood. Partial or total deafness may result from sclerosis in the middle ear or pressure on the auditory nerve. The other cranial nerves are rarely involved, and increased intracranial pressure is not a problem. Habitus and general health are normal and neither skeletal fragility nor dyshaemopoesis occurs.

The clinical features and complications in 15 individuals in five generations of a British-South African kindred have been reviewed by Beighton et al. (1979).

Radiographic Manifestations

Sclerosis of the skull and widening of the metaphyses of the tubular bones are the main radiographic features. The changes are age-related and vary in severity from one patient to another. The radiographic manifestations have been reviewed by Holt (1966), and Spiro et al. (1975).

Skull

The skull vault and base are sclerotic, with mild hyperostosis. Sclerosis may be particularly evident along suture lines, and the mastoid and paranasal air sinuses are often obliterated. Paranasal bone overgrowth gives a radiological appearance of hypertelorism. The mandible may be prominent and asymmetrical.

Spine

The spine is normal.

Chest and Pelvis

Modelling of the medial portions of the clavicles and costochondral junction is mildly defective. The pelvis is normal.

Limbs

The metaphyses of the long bones are widened, with cortical thinning, and they present a club-shaped configuration. This is particularly evident in the lower end of the femur. The carpus and tarsus are normal but mild under-modelling is evident in the tubular bones of the extremities. It is noteworthy

Table 7-1. Clinical and radiological features of Pyle disease and the craniometaphyseal dysplasias

	Pyle disease	CMD AD type	CMD AR type
Reported cases	20+	50+	10
Clinical features			
Facial distortion	–	+	+++
Cranial nerve palsy	–	+	++
Bone fragility	+	–	–
Radiographic features			
Cranial sclerosis	+	++	+++
Modelling defects in long bones	+++	+	+
Configuration of distal femora	Erlenmeyer flask	Club-shaped	Club-shaped

that the bone ends in adults with CMD are club-shaped, whereas in childhood they have the Erlenmeyer flask appearance generally associated with Pyle disease.

Comment

The autosomal recessive type of CMD is rare: fewer than ten case reports can be recognised in the literature. The clinical changes are severe, with enlargement of the skull, distortion of the mandible, and marked paranasal and glabellar bossing. The teeth are irregular and carious, deafness and facial palsy are common, and compression of the optic nerves may occur. Radiographically, the skull is sclerotic and hyperostotic, with obliteration of the sinuses and bony encroachment upon the cranial foramina. The archaic designation 'leontiasis ossea' has been applied to at least one affected individual on the basis of these changes. The spine and the pelvis are uninvolved and the changes in the long bones resemble those of the common autosomal dominant type of CMD.

Although the manifestations of the autosomal dominant type of CMD are variable, diagnosis is not difficult. Confusion between dominant and recessive CMD and Pyle disease (see Chap. 6) is based upon semantic problems rather than the actual clinical or radiological situation. Distinguishing clinical and radiographic features are listed in Table 7-1.

References

BEIGHTON P, HORAN F, HAMERSMA H (1977) A review of the osteopetroses. Postgrad Med J 53:507

BEIGHTON P, HAMERSMA H, HORAN F (1979) Craniometaphyseal dysplasia. Variability of expression within a large family. Clin Genet 15:252

GARCIN M, CAGNOT C, MAGNAN J (1975) La dysplasie cranio-metaphysaire de Pyle. Une nouvelle observation. J Fr Otorhinolaryngol 24:119

GORLIN RJ, SPRANGER J, KOSZALKA MF (1969) Genetic craniotubular bone dysplasias and hyperostoses. A critical analysis. Birth Defects 5/4:79

HOLT JF (1966) The evolution of cranio-metaphyseal dysplasia. Ann Radiol (Paris) 9:109

JACKSON WPU, ALBRIGHT F, DREWRY G, HANELIN J, RUBIN ML (1954) Metaphyseal dysplasia, epiphyseal dysplasia, diaphyseal dysplasia and related conditions. Arch Intern Med 94/6:871

LEHMANN ECH (1957) Familial osteodystrophy of the skull and face. J Bone Joint Surg [Br] 39:313

LIEVRE JA, FISCHGOLD DH (1956) Leontiasis ossea chez l'enfant (osteopetrose partielle probable). Presse Méd 64:763

MARTIN FW (1977) Craniometaphyseal dysplasia. J Laryngol Otol 91:159

MILLARD DR, MAISELS DD, BATSONE JHF, YATES BW (1967) Craniofacial surgery in craniometaphyseal dysplasia. Am J Surg 113:615

MORI PA, HOLT JF (1956) Cranial manifestations of familial metaphyseal dysplasia. Radiology 66:335

ROSS MW, ALTMAN DH (1967) Familial metaphyseal dysplasia. Review of the clinical and radiologic features of Pyle's disease. Clin Pediatr 63:143

SPIRO PC, HAMERSMA H, BEIGHTON P (1975) Radiology of the autosomal dominant form of craniometaphyseal dysplasia. S Afr Med J 49:839

SPRANGER J, PAULSEN J, LEHMANN W (1965) Die kraniometaphysaere Dysplasie (Pyle). Z Kinderheilk 93:64

STOOL SE, CARUSO VG (1973) Cranial metaphyseal dysplasia. Arch Otolaryngol 97:410

The spectrum of this condition is demonstrated by a family study which principally involves a grandmother, son, and granddaughter. The skeletal survey of the son emphasises the fact that the main abnormalities are in the skull and long bones. Skull radiographs of other adult relatives are also presented to illustrate the range of cranial involvement

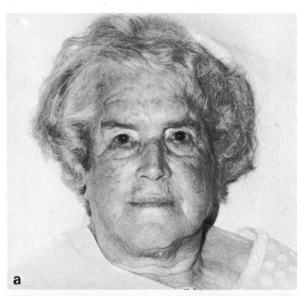

Case I
Grandmother, aged 74 years

Fig. 7-1. (a) The jaw is prominent but the face is otherwise normal

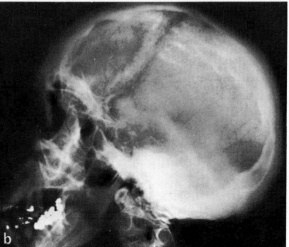

Fig. 7-1. (b) Skull. Basal sclerosis and hyperostosis is particularly marked in the occipital region (Beighton et al. 1979)

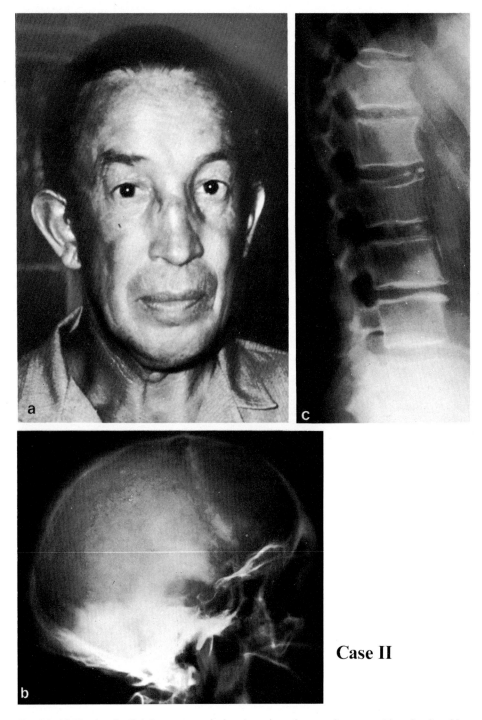

Fig. 7-2. (a) The jaw is slightly asymmetrical and a minor degree of paranasal bossing is evident (Beighton et al. 1979). (b) Skull. Lateral view showing sclerosis in the base and vault and along the coronal suture. (c) Spine. Degenerative changes are present but the vertebrae are not sclerotic

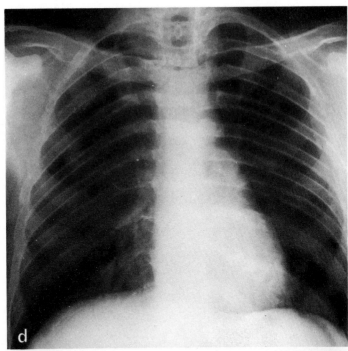

Fig. 7-2. (d) Chest. The clavicles are widened but not sclerotic

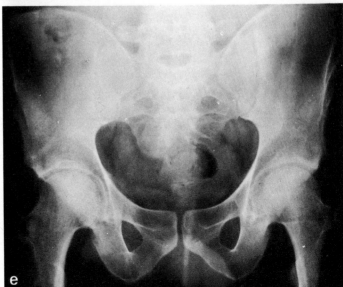

Fig. 7-2. (e) Pelvis. No sclerosis. Coxa vara of minor degree and underdevelopment of the iliac wings are evident

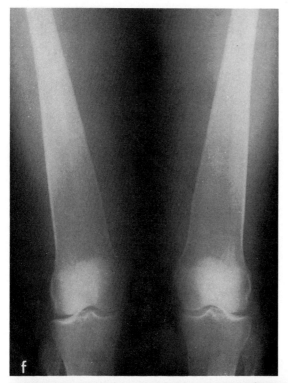

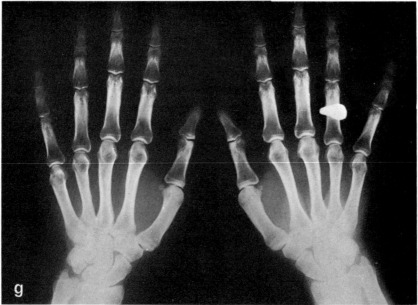

Fig. 7-2. (f) Knees. The metaphyses show 'club-shaped' undermodelling. (g) Hands. Mild cortical thickening is present in the phalanges

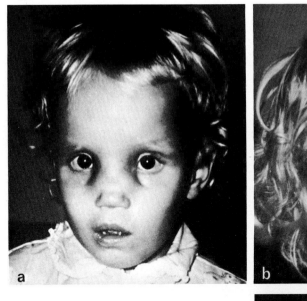
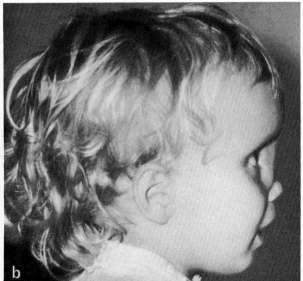
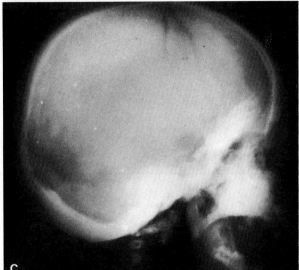

Case III
Granddaughter aged 3 years

Fig. 7-3. (a and b) Paranasal bossing is very obvious (Beighton et al. 1979). (c) Skull. Mild sclerosis is present in the base and calvarium (Spiro et al. 1975)

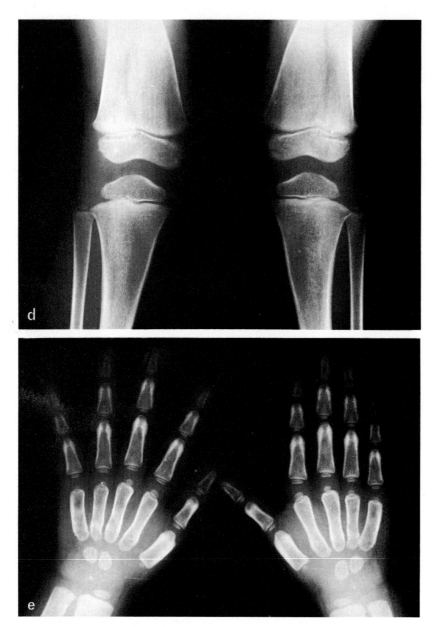

Fig. 7-3. (d) Knees. Metaphyseal modelling is defective. At this stage the lower femora are flask-shaped but by adulthood they will have a 'club' configuration (Beighton et al. 1977). (e) Hands. Slight undermodelling and cortical thickening is seen in the phalanges (Spiro et al. 1975)

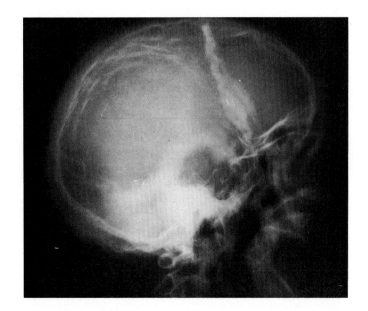

Case IV
Brother of Patient 2, aged 43 years

Fig. 7-4. Skull. Sclerosis of occipital region and major sutures

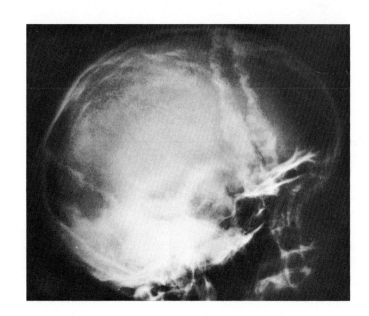

Case V
Sister of Patient 2, aged 47 years

Fig. 7-5. Skull. Sclerosis of the base and sutures is similar to that seen in her adult siblings (Spiro et al. 1975)

Chapter 8

Craniodiaphyseal Dysplasia

Historical and Nosological Considerations

JOSEPH et al. (1958) reported a patient with severe sclerosis of the skull, cited a similar case from HALLIDAY (1949), and termed the disorder 'dysplasie craniodiaphysaire progressive.' At this time the condition was thought to be related to CAMURATI-ENGELMANN disease.

In their critical review of genetic craniotubular bone dysplasias and hyperostoses GORLIN et al. (1969) defined craniodiaphyseal dysplasia (CDD) as a very severe bone dysplasia characterised by massive hyperostosis and sclerosis, involving the skull and facial bones especially. In earlier reports a number of affected individuals with gross distortion of the facies can be identified in patients grouped under the non-specific designation 'leontiasis ossea.' Examples of this situation include reports of DE SOUZA (1927), GEMMELL (1935), and STRANSKY et al. (1962).

MACPHERSON (1974) presented case details of three children with CDD and pointed out that there were considerable discrepancies in their manifestations and that some overlapped with other craniotubular dysplasias and hyperostoses. The investigator went on to make the very reasonable suggestion that CDD might be a group of diseases rather than a single entity.

In recent reports KAITILA et al. (1975) drew attention to the importance of nasal and lacrimal obstruction in CDD, while TUCKER et al. (1976) emphasised the progressive nature of the condition and described the evolution of the radiographic changes.

Clinical Features

CDD is a progressive disorder in which distortion of the face becomes apparent in early childhood. Due to bony overgrowth the head circumference may be increased, and marked paranasal bossing, flattening of the nasal bridge and malformation of the nasal cartilages are major features. The changes in the nose are of much greater magnitude than in the other craniotubular dysplasias, and obstruction of the nasal airways and lacrimal ducts may be a presenting feature in infancy. Compression of the second and eighth cranial nerves has led to blindness and deafness in some patients, while mental retardation, epilepsy, and stunted growth are other complications which have been reported.

Radiographic Manifestations

In the fully developed case, the great severity of the involvement of the skull distinguishes CDD from other similar disorders. Descriptions of changes in the diaphyses of the tubular bones and other sites have varied from patient to patient, reflecting diagnostic uncertainty and nosological confusion. This situation has been discussed in detail from the radiological standpoint by MACPHERSON (1974) and TUCKER et al. (1976).

Skull

The whole skull, including the mandible and facial bones, shows progressive hyperostosis and sclerosis, with defective aeration of the sinuses and occlusion of the nasal passages. Progressive bony overgrowth leads to dental malocclusion and entrapment of cranial nerves. Ultimately the skull is massively thickened and distorted.

Spine

Changes in the spine are inconsistent and may approach normality. Severe sclerosis of the vertebral arches contrasting with mild to moderate changes in the vertebral bodies has been stressed in some reports.

Chest and Pelvis

The clavicles, ribs and pelvis show varying degrees of sclerosis and hyperostosis, but involvement at these sites is not a major feature.

Limbs

The tubular bones show diaphyseal endosteal cortical thickening and defective modelling. In younger patients, the expansion of the diaphyses gives a straight 'policeman's nightstick' appearance to the bones. The short cylindrical bones of the hands may be affected in a similar fashion. These changes are variable in degree and distribution, and in some patients they have regressed with the passage of time. In all instances the involvement of the long bones is overshadowed by gross changes in the skull.

Comment

Although only about ten patients with CDD have been reported, it is likely that the condition is heterogeneous. The occurrence in a brother and sister (DE SOUZA 1927) and a mention of parental consanguinity (HALLIDAY 1949) are consistent with autosomal recessive inheritance, and it is probable that all forms are transmitted by this mechanism.

At a radiological level, a mild case of CDD, may be difficult to distinguish from CAMURATI-ENGELMANN disease. However, involvement of the short tubular bones and the flat bones in the former condition are important diagnostic pointers. In the fully developed severe form of CDD, the gross facial changes are unlike any other condition. The distinguishing features of craniodiaphyseal dysplasia and CAMURATI-ENGELMANN disease are listed in Table 14-1.

References

DE SOUZA O (1927) Leontiasis ossea. Case reports. Porto Alegre Fac Med 13:47

GEMMELL JH (1935) Leontiasis ossea: A clinical and roentgenological entity: Report of a case. Radiology 25:723

GORLIN RJ, SPRANGER J. KOSZALKA MF (1969) Genetic craniotubular bone dysplasias and hyperostoses: A critical analysis. Birth Defects 5/4:79

HALLIDAY J (1949) A rare case of bone dystrophy. Br J Surg 37:52

JOSEPH R, LEFEBVRE J, GUY E, JOB JC (1958) Dysplasie craniodiayphysaire progressive. Ann Radiol (Paris) 1:477

KAITILA I, STEWART RE, LANDOW E, LACHMAN R, RIMOIN DL (1975) Craniodiaphyseal dysplasia. Birth Defects 11/6:359

MACPHERSON RI (1974) Craniodiaphyseal dysplasia, a disease or group of diseases? J Can Assoc Radiol 25:2

STRANSKY E, MABILANGAN I, LARA RT (1962) On Paget's disease with leontiasis ossea and hypothreosis starting in early childhood. Ann Pediatr 199:393

TUCKER AS, KLEIN L, ANTONY GJ (1976) Craniodiaphyseal dysplasia: Evolution over a five-year period. Skeletal Radiol. 1:47

This case is presented by courtesy of Dr Arthur S. Tucker of the University Hospital, Cleveland, U.S.A.
The progression over a five-year period illustrates some of the dilemmas which arise in this condition.
This patient was initially considered to have Engelmann's disease, but following the development of sclerosis
in the skull the diagnosis was changed to craniodiaphyseal dysplasia (Tucker et al. 1976)

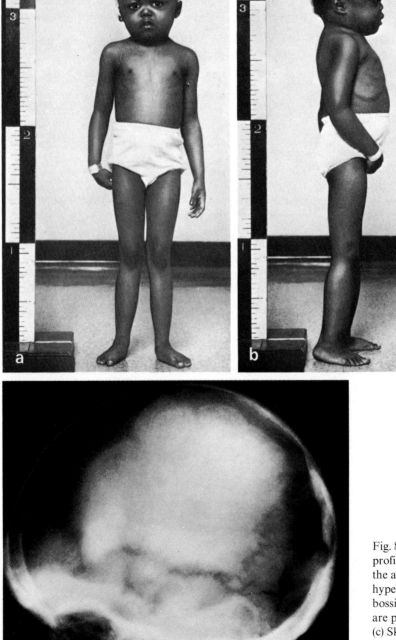

Fig. 8-1. (a and b) Frontal and
profile appearance of the patient at
the age of 4 years, showing mild
hypertelorism and marked frontal
bossing. Minor valgus deformities
are present at the knees.
(c) Skull at $1^1/_2$ years. Sclerosis
is present in the parietal bones and
the base

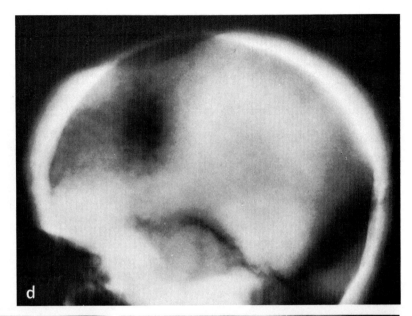

Fig. 8-1. (d) Skull at 4 years. Diffuse sclerosis of the calvarium is now evident

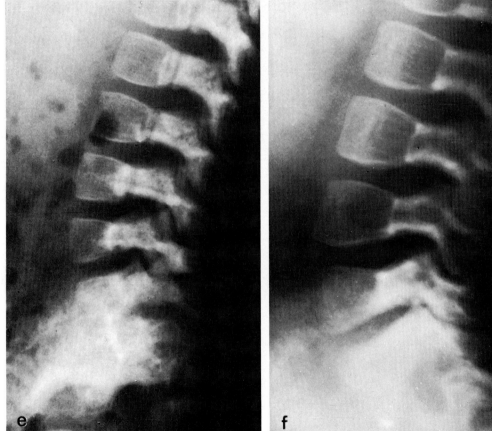

Fig. 8-1. (e) Spine, lumbosacral region at 1¹/₂ years. The vertebral bodies are normal, but the neural arches are sclerotic

Fig. 8-1. (f) Three years later, differential density between the bodies and neural arches is still present but less striking

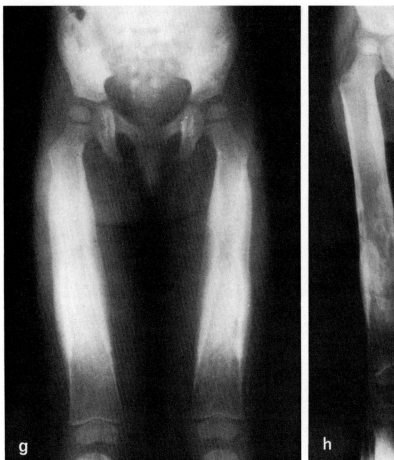
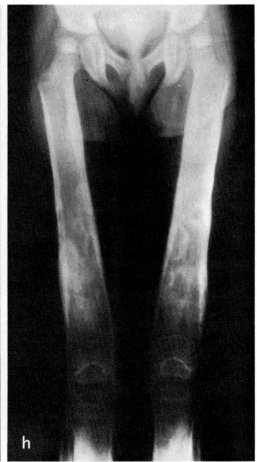

Fig. 8-1. (g) Femora at $1^1/_2$ years demonstrating marked diaphyseal cortical thickening

Fig. 8-1. (h) Three years later the shafts are thick and undermodelled. Localised cortical thickening creates a whorled pattern

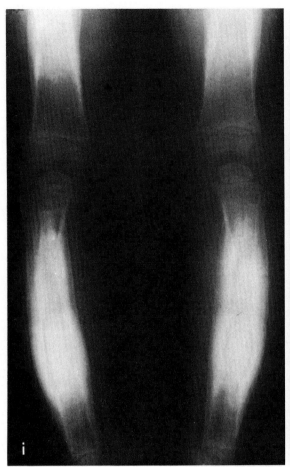

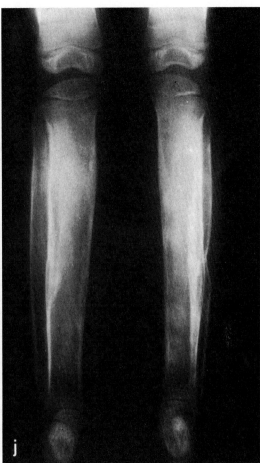

Fig. 8-1. (i) Tibiae at $1\frac{1}{2}$ years. These bones are fusiform with slight lateral bowing. The mid-shaft cortices are sclerotic and moderately thickened

Fig. 8-1. (j) Three years later the tibiae and fibulae are cylindrical. The cortices are generally thin but moderate irregular thickening persists

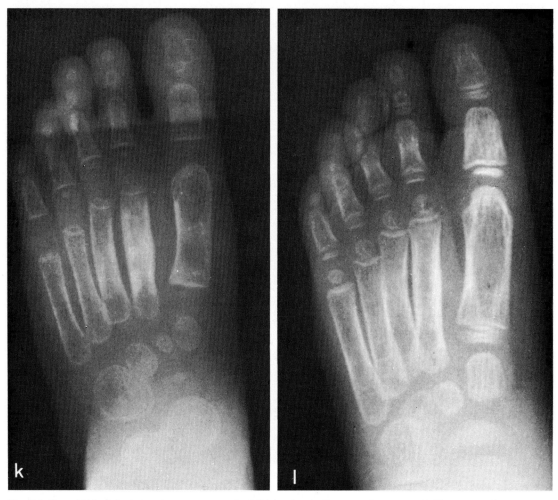

Fig. 8-1. (k and l) Left foot showing uneven cortical thickening in the second metatarsal. Three years later it is still present but less pronounced

Chapter 9

Frontometaphyseal Dysplasia

Historical and Nosological Considerations

Frontometaphyseal dysplasia (FMD) was delineated by GORLIN and COHEN (1969) when they described the association of a prominent supra-orbital ridge with defective skeletal modelling and deafness. The range of manifestations was expanded by DANKS et al. (1972), HOLT et al. (1972), DANKS and MAYNE (1974), and ARENBERG et al. (1974). Subsequently, SAUVEGRAIN et al. (1975) tabulated the clinical and radiographic features of eight patients, while the orthopaedic complications were reviewed by KLEINSORGE and BOTTGER (1977) and MEDLAR and CRAWFORD (1978).

The familial nature of FMD became apparent when JERVIS and JENKINS (1975) reported affected half-brothers, and WEISS et al. (1976) and KASSNER et al. (1976) described affected sons with mildly affected mothers.

Retrospectively, the diagnosis of FMD can be suspected in the young woman with a marked supra-orbital prominence reported by LISCHI (1967) and in the young man described by WALKER (1969) as a possible example of craniometaphyseal or diaphyseal dysplasia. Conversely, the 19-year-old male described by SCHEEPER (1967) and sometimes quoted as a case of FMD was probably unaffected.

About 15 patients have now been reported, but this figure is not strictly accurate as a number of individuals have featured in more than one publication. Details are shown in Table 9-1.

Clinical Features

A visor-like prominence of the supra-orbital ridge is evident in early childhood. The mandible is constricted anteriorly, and dental irregularities may result in malocclusion. Height is normal but the limbs are long in proportion to the trunk. The tibiae are curved backwards and mild valgus deformities are present in the knees. The elbows lack full extension and rotation, and the digits are progressively flexed. Other, less consistent musculoskeletal features include muscle wasting and scoliosis.

Table 9-1. Previous reports of frontometaphyseal dysplasia

	Sex	Age	Country of origin	Comment
LISCHI (1967)	F	13	Italy	Diagnosed as CMD Description fits FMD
WALKER (1969)	M	31	U.S.A.	Diagnosed as CDD or CMD Illustrations show definite FMD
GORLIN and COHEN (1969)	M	19	U.S.A.	First definitive case description
DANKS et al. (1972)	M	12	Australia (Italian stock)	Progressive digital deformities emphasised
HOLT et al. (1972)	M	18	U.S.A.	Pattern profile analysis
	F	13	U.S.A.	Differential diagnosis reviewed
STERN et al. (1972)	M	21		Previously reported by Holt et al. (1972)
	F	17		Ocular and cosmetic problems reviewed
ARENBERG et al. (1974)	M	22		Previously reported by Holt et al. (1972) ENT complications discussed
DANKS and MAYNE (1974)	M	15		Previously reported by Danks et al. (1972)
SAUVEGRAIN et al. (1975)	M	11	France	Mental retardation
JERVIS and JENKINS (1975)	M	18	U.S.A. (negro)	Half-brothers with severe mental retardation
	M	22		X-linked inheritance suggested
KASSNER et al. (1976)	M	8	U.S.A. (mixed ancestry)	AD inheritance with variable expression suggested
	M	23		Previously reported by Jervis and Jenkins (1975)
	M	17		
WEISS et al. (1976)	M	10	U.S.A.	Mother mildly affected Dominant inheritance proposed
VON KLEINSORGE and BÖTTGER (1977)	F	16	Germany	Manifestations tabulated
MEDLAR and CRAWFORD (1978)	M	13	U.S.A.	Orthopaedic problems reviewed

Mixed deafness is a common complication, although it may be delayed until middle age. The cranial nerves are otherwise uninvolved, and in all but three reported patients, intelligence has been normal.

Radiographic Manifestations

The prominent supra-orbital ridge and widespread but mild modelling defects are the main radiological features. These have been reviewed and tabulated by HOLT et al. (1972), SAUVEGRAIN et al. (1975), KASSNER et al. (1976) and von KLEINSORGE and BOTTGER (1977).

Skull

The skull is rectangular in shape, with a 'helmet' appearance and there is gross overgrowth and hyperostosis of the supra-orbital ridge. Sclerosis of the rest of the calvarium is patchy and variable in extent, but the paranasal sinuses are poorly developed. The foramen magnum may be large. The mandible is underdeveloped, with anterior constriction, and dental anomalies may be evident.

Spine

A variety of structural defects may be present in the cervical spine, including fusions and subluxations, an anomalous position of the odontoid process and absence of the posterior arch of the atlas. Thoracic and lumbar vertebral bodies are somewhat flattened and dysplastic and spinal malalignment may be present.

Chest and Pelvis

The posterior portions of the ribs are thin and irregular in contour. There is some constriction of the base of the iliac bones, with intrapelvic protrusion of the acetabula and flaring of the iliac wings.

Limbs

The skeleton is generally dysplastic, with mild undertubulation of the metaphyses of all long bones. The femoral necks are expanded and mild coxa valga is evident. The tibia and fibula are wavy and bowed backwards.
In the hands, the metacarpals and phalanges are elongated and expanded with narrowing of the joint spaces. The bones of the carpus may be fused and eroded. Similar changes are seen in the feet.

Comment

The combination of a marked supra-orbital ridge and mild generalised skeletal modelling defects serves to distinguish FMD from the other craniotubular dysplasias. Osteodysplasty (see Chap. 10) and FMD have many features in common, and it is possible that some reported patients with the former condition were in fact suffering from FMD. Indeed, FMD and osteodysplasty might transpire to be the same entity but at present this remains a matter of speculation.

FMD might be heterogeneous, with the existence of distinct autosomal dominant and X-linked types. So far these have not been clearly delineated and the available evidence favours the latter mode of inheritance (BEIGHTON and HAMERSMA 1980).

DANKS et al. (1972) and WEISS et al. (1976) have demonstrated metachromasia in cultured fibroblasts in some affected individuals. This finding is of potential value in terms of settling the question of heterogeneity and exploring the relationship between FMD and osteodysplasty.

References

ARENBERG IK, SHAMBAUGH GE, VALVASSORI GE (1974) Otolaryngologic manifestations of frontometaphyseal dysplasia. Arch Otolaryngol 99:52

BEIGHTON P, HAMERSMA H (1980) Frontometaphyseal dysplasia: Autosomal dominant or X-linked? J Med Genet 17:53

DANKS DM, MAYNE V (1974) Frontometaphyseal dysplasia: A progressive disease of bone and connective tissue. Birth Defects 10/12:57

DANKS DM, MAYNE V, HALL RK, McKINNON MC (1972) Fronto-metaphyseal dysplasia. Am J Dis Child 123:254

GORLIN RJ, COHEN MM (1969) Frontometaphyseal dysplasia. Am J Dis Child 118:487

HOLT JF, THOMPSON GR, ARENBERG IK (1972) Frontometaphyseal dysplasia. Radiol Clin North Am 10/2:225

JERVIS GA, JENKINS EC (1975) Case report 31. Syndrome Identification 3/1:18

KASSNER EG, HALLER JO, REDDY VH, MITAROTUNDO A, KATZ I (1976) Frontometaphyseal dysplasia: Evidence for autosomal dominant inheritance. A J R 127:927

KLEINSORGE H, BOTTGER E (1977) Das Gorlin-Cohen-Syndrom (fronto-metaphysäre Dysplasia). Fortschr Roentgenstr 127:451

LISCHI G (1967) Le torus supraorbitalis (variation cranienne rare). J Radiol Electrol Med Nucl 48:463

MEDLAR RC, CRAWFORD AH (1978) Frontometaphyseal dysplasia presenting as scoliosis: A report of a family with four cases. J Bone Joint Surg 60:392

POZNANSKI AK, GARN SM, NAGY JM, GALL JC (1972) Metacarpophalangeal profile patterns in the evaluation of skeletal malformations. Radiology 104/1:1

SAUVEGRAIN J. LOMBARD M, GAREL L, TRUSCELLI D (1975) Dysplasie fronto-metaphysaire. Ann Radiol (Paris) 18/2:155

SCHEEPER JH (1967) A patient with skeletal abnormalities due to dysplasia and hypoplasia of the muscular system. Radiol Clin North Am 36:339

STERN SD, ARENBERG IK, ONEAL RM, SANDALL GS, HOLT JF (1972) The ocular and cosmetic problems in frontometaphyseal dysplasia. J Pediatr Ophthalmol 9/3:151

WALKER BA (1969) A craniodiaphyseal dysplasia or craniometaphyseal dysplasia? Type. Birth Defects 5:298

WEISS L, REYNOLDS WA, SZYMANOWSKI RT (1976) Frontometaphyseal dysplasia. Am J Dis Child 130:259

The features of the condition are illustrated by a series of radiographs of a 44-year-old male who is the oldest recorded patient with frontometaphyseal dysplasia. This case is presented by kind permission of Professor H. Hamersma of the University of Pretoria (Beighton and Hamersma 1980)

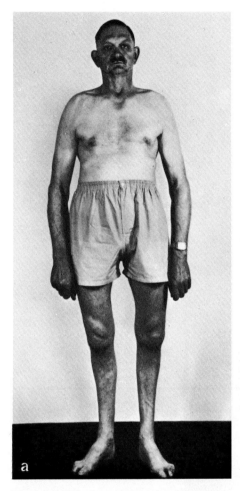

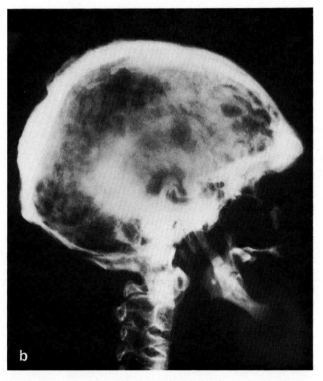

Fig. 9-1. (a) The brow is prominent and the mandible is narrow anteriorly. The limbs are disproportionately long, and tibia recurvatum is present. The digits show flexion deformities

Fig. 9-1. (b) Skull. Prominence of the supra-orbital ridge is a major feature of the condition. Irregular sclerosis is present throughout the skull and in this patient is exceptionally severe, possibly due to age. The changes in the skull were initially misdiagnosed as Paget disease

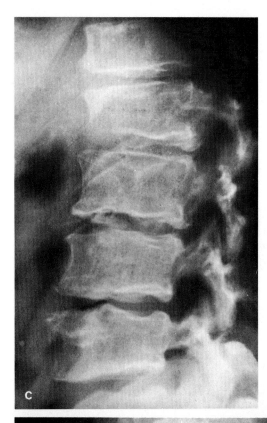

Fig. 9-1. (c) Spine.
Platyspondyly,
irregularity of disc
spaces and associated
degenerative changes
are seen

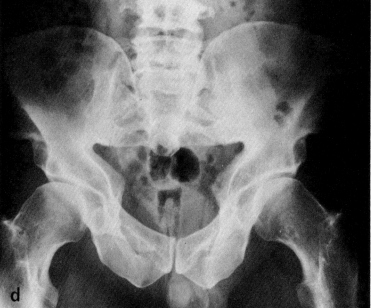

Fig. 9-1. (d) Pelvis. Protrusio acetabuli and narrowing of the obturator
foramina distort the pelvic inlet. The ilia are flared

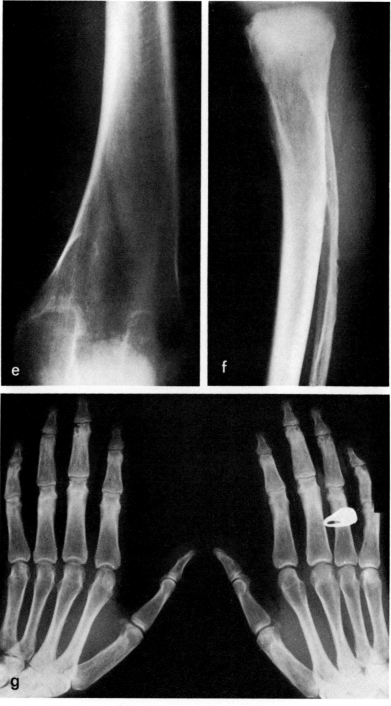

Fig. 9-1. (e) Distal femora showing mild undermodelling. (f) Leg. The tibia and fibula are curved posterolaterally. (g) Hand. The phalanges show marked undermodelling and disproportion in length. Erosions are present in the distal interphalangeal joints

Chapter 10

Osteodysplasty
(Melnick-Needles Syndrome)

Historical and Nosological Considerations

MELNICK and NEEDLES (1966) described two unrelated kindreds in the
U.S.A. in which at least 13 persons had an 'undiagnosed bone dysplasia.'
COSTE et al. (1968) recognised a 50-year-old female with identical features
and coined the term 'osteodysplasty' for the condition. This designation
was derived from the Greek and was intended to convey the meaning 'badly
formed.' This woman, together with an affected 7-month-old girl, was reported again in the French literature by the same authors (MAROTEAUX et
al. 1968).

The range of clinical and radiographic features has been expanded in sub-
sequent reports, although in view of possible overlap with frontometaphyseal dysplasia (see Chap. 9) these should be interpreted with caution.
Details of reported cases are listed in Table 10-1.

Clinical Features

The patients mentioned in the earlier reports bore a strong facial resemblance to each other. Their facial features included bulging eyes, prominent
cheeks and nose, high foreheads, malaligned teeth, and small chins. Their
general health was good, although ear infections were common. The limbs
showed some bowing and the distal phalanges were short. Some had important complications, such as dislocation of the hips and kyphoscoliosis,
while others were recognised only on radiographic survey of the affected
kindreds.

In more recent case descriptions, additional manifestations have included
pectus excavatum, pulmonary hypertension, marrow hypoplasia and obstructive uropathy. It must be emphasised, however, that in the majority of
individuals in the original kindreds studied by MELNICK and NEEDLES (1966)
the condition was comparatively benign.

Table 10-1. Reported cases of osteodysplasty

Author	Patient	Country of origin	Comments
MELNICK and NEEDLES (1966)	13 patients in two kindreds	U.S.A. (Hungarian-Italian Anglo-Saxon)	
COSTE et al. (1968)	Female, 50	France	Designation "osteodysplasty" proposed
MAROTEAUX et al. (1968)	Female, 50 (same patient as above)	France	Dominant inheritance suggested
MARTIN et al. (1971)	Female, newborn	France	Multiple abnormalities evident at birth
GRUMBACH et al. (1974)	Female, 26	France	X-ray review
LEIBER and HÖVELS (1975)	Female, 8	Germany	Clinical and radiographic features reviewed
WENDLER and KELLERER (1975)	Female, 6	Austria	Radiography reviewed
MOADEL and BRYK (1977)	Female, 4	U.S.A.	Died following operation for pectus excavatum
KLINT et al. (1977)	Female, $3^{1}/_{2}$	U.S.A.	Pulmonary hypertension. Marrow hyperplasia
GORLIN and LANGER (1978)	Female, 18 Female, 20 Female, 44 with two affected daughters	U.S.A. Holland U.S.A.	X-ray changes in mandible noted

Radiographic Manifestations

The diagnosis is reached by recognition of the typical facies and the widespread radiographic changes. Although there is sclerosis in the skull and metaphyseal deformities with irregularities of cortical density, the major consistent feature is the presence of 'badly formed' elements, which are most prominent in the mandible, thoracic cage and pelvic girdle. Changes in the ribs and long bones permitted radiographic diagnosis in the fetus of an affected mother at 6 months' gestation. (MELNICK and NEEDLES 1966).

Skull

The base of the skull is sclerotic and the mastoid sinuses are obliterated. Closure of the anterior fontanelle is delayed. Micrognathia results from hypoplasia of the horizontal rami of the mandible. The mandibular angle is rounded and the coronoid processes are small. Cystic changes have been noted in the mandible (GORLIN and LANGER 1978).

Spine

There are no remarkable abnormalities in the spine, but scoliosis and kyphosis may occur, with some increased height and scalloping of vertebral bodies and decrease in disc spaces.

Chest and Pelvis

Characteristic features are seen in these regions. The ribs are distorted, with irregularities and narrowing which give them a ribbon-like appearance. The clavicles have accentuation of their sigmoid shape, and pectus excavatum may be present.

In the pelvis the ischial and pubic bones are hypoplastic, so that the obturator foramina and acetabular regions are flattened. The iliac wings are flared and the crests may appear grooved when seen longitudinally.

Limbs

The long bones have mild metaphyseal flaring and bowing. Contour alterations rather than changes in cortical density predominate. The upper femora show a sudden deviation of their longitudinal axes, which is associated with pronounced coxa vara (FAURÉ 1978). The humeri are bowed posteriorly and the tibiae may be curved, with lateral bowing.

The bones of the hands and feet are relatively normal apart from some distal shortening which is most marked in the terminal phalanges of the thumbs and great toes.

Comment

There is controversy concerning the syndromic indentity of osteodysplasty and its relationship with frontometaphyseal dysplasia (see Chap. 9). MAROTEAUX (1974) contended that these conditions were the result of variation in phenotypic expression of the same abnormal gene; GORLIN et al. (1976) considered that they were distinct entities. In this context it is remarkable that, apart from the members of the original families reported by MELNICK and NEEDLES (1966), virtually every patient with osteodysplasty has been a female. Conversely, nearly every description of frontometaphyseal dysplasia has concerned a male.

There is certainly overlap in the stigmata of these two conditions, and in the absence of any objective marker firm diagnosis is not always easy. In view of this confusion, it is possible that some reports of osteodysplasty have concerned frontometaphyseal dysplasia, and vice versa: a young deaf patient with severe skeletal problemes described by SELLARS and BEIGHTON (1978) might be an example of this situation.

Other Forms of Osteodysplasia

Inheritance in the original kindreds reported by MELNICK and NEEDLES (1966) was autosomal dominant, and the 'autosomal recessive precocious type of osteodysplasia' delineated by KOZLOWSKI et al. (1973), which is lethal in infancy, is clearly a distinct entity. HANSON et al. (1977) described a seven-year-old child with a syndrome of craniofacial anomalies, ectodermal defects, and chondro-osseous dysplasia which resembled the Melnick-Needles syndrome. This is also likely to be a separate disorder.

Familial osteodysplasia (ANDERSON et al. 1972; BUCHIGNANI et al. 1972) in which the major feature is abnormal mandibular development has nothing more than a semantic relationship with the osteodysplasty of MELNICK and NEEDLES.

References

COSTE F, MAROTEAUX P, CHOURAKI L (1968) Osteodysplasty (Melnick and Needles syndrome): Report of a case. Ann Rheum Dis 27:360

GORLIN RJ, LANGER LO (1978) Melnick-Needles syndrome: Radiographic alterations in the mandible. Radiology 128:351

GORLIN RJ, PINDBORG JJ, COHEN MM (1976) In: Syndromes of the head and neck, 2nd edn. McGraw-Hill, New York

GRUMBACH Y, PIUSSAN C, RÉMOND A, ROZAN R, TRINEZ G (1974) Etude radiologique d'un cas d'ostéodysplastie. J Radiol Electrol Méd Nucl 55:129

KLINT RB, AGUSTSSON MH, McALISTER WH (1977) Melnick-Needles osteodysplasia associated with pulmonary hypertension, obstructive uropathy and marrow hypoplasia. Pediatr Radiol 6:49

LEIBER B, HÖVELS O (1975) Melnick-Needles syndrom. Monatsschrift Kinderheilkd 123:178

MARTIN C, BABIN J-P, KAUFFMANN J-M, FONTAN D, MICHEAU M (1971) Un cas d'ostéodysplasie (syndrome de Melnick et de Needles). Arch Fr Pédiatr 28:446

MAROTEAUX P, CHOURAKI L, COSTE F (1968) L'ostéodysplastie (syndrome de Melnick et de Needles). Presse Méd 76:715

MAROTEAUX P (1974) In: Maladies osseuses de l'enfant. Flammarion, Paris, p 148

MELNICK JC, NEEDLES CF (1966) An undiagnosed bone dysplasia: A 2 family study of 4 generations and 3 generations. A J R 97:39

MOADEL E, BRYK D (1977) Radiological quiz. Radiology 123:154

SELLARS SL, BEIGHTON PH (1978) Deafness in osteodysplasty of Melnick and Needles. Arch Otolaryngol 104:225

WENDLER H, KELLERER K (1975) Osteodysplasie Syndrom (Melnick Needles). Fortschr Roentgenstr 122:309

References – Other Forms of Osteodysplasia

ANDERSON LG, COOK AJ, COCCARO PJ, CORO CJ, BOSMA JF (1972) Familial osteodysplasia. J A M A 220:1687

BUCHIGNANI JS, COOK AJ, ANDERSON LG (1972) Roentgenographic findings in familial osteodysplasia. A J R 116:602

HANSON JW, GRAHAM CB, HALL JG (1977) A syndrome of craniofacial anomalies, ectodermal defects and chondro-osseous dysplasia with similarities to Melnick-Needles syndrome. Birth Defects 13/3B:243

KOZLOWSKI K, MAYNE V, DANKS DM (1973) Precocious type of osteodysplasia. A new autosomal recessive form. Acta Radiol (Stockh) 14:171

There is controversy concerning the relationship between osteodysplasty and frontometaphyseal dysplasia, and some experts believe that they are the same condition. Case 1 is the proband of the first kindred reported by Melnick and Needles (1966). Radiographs 10-1a, b, c, d appeared in the original article and were obtained at the age of 3 years. These films and further views taken at 13 years are depicted by courtesy of Dr John Melnick of Youngstown, Ohio. Considerable progression of the disorder taken place in this ten-year period. Case 2, a 12-year-old boy, has features of both osteodysplasty and frontometaphyseal dysplasia

Case I

Girl aged 3 years (Fig. 10-1a to 10-1d) and at the age of 13 (Fig. 10-1e–h)

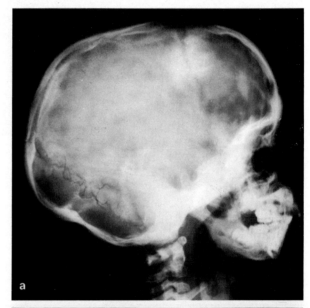

Fig. 10-1. (a) Skull at 3 years of age. The base is sclerotic and the mandible is small (Melnick and Needles 1966)

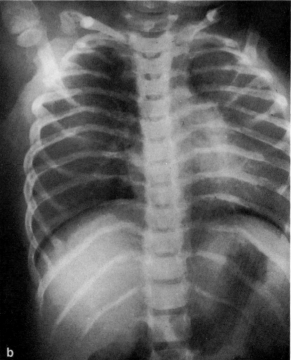

Fig. 10-1. (b) Chest at 3 years of age. Cortical irregularities of the ribs produces a ribbon-like appearance (Melnick and Needles 1966)

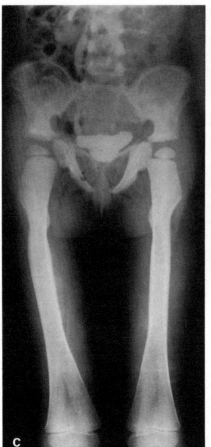

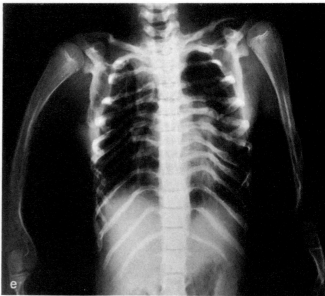

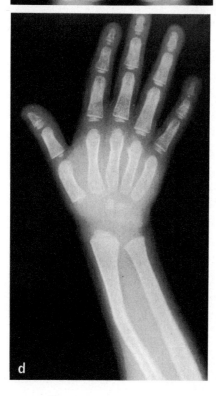

Fig. 10-1. (c) Pelvis and femora at 3 years of age. The iliac bones show flaring of their crests and flattening of the acetabula. Coxa valga and metaphyseal widening are present in the femora. These films were part of an IVP series and a hydro-ureter is demonstrated (Melnick and Needles 1966). (d) Hand and forearm at 3 years of age. The terminal phalanges of the thumbs are short, the metacarpals are undermodelled, and the radius is bowed (Melnick and Needles 1966). (e) Chest at 13 years of age. The thorax is deformed and the ribs are very irregular

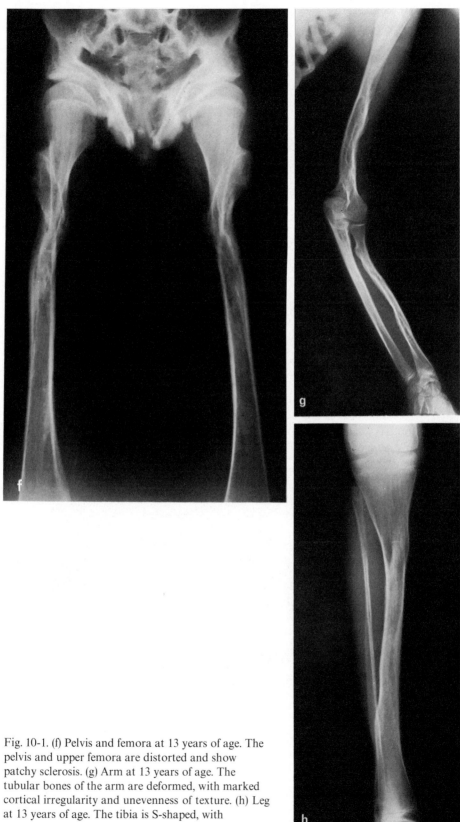

Fig. 10-1. (f) Pelvis and femora at 13 years of age. The pelvis and upper femora are distorted and show patchy sclerosis. (g) Arm at 13 years of age. The tubular bones of the arm are deformed, with marked cortical irregularity and unevenness of texture. (h) Leg at 13 years of age. The tibia is S-shaped, with moderate metaphyseal flaring

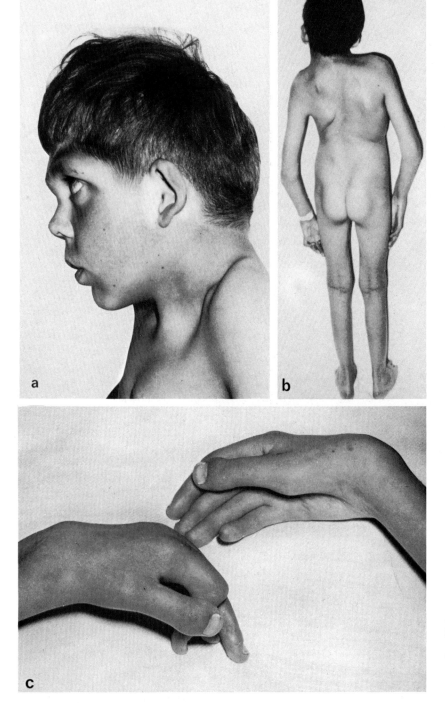

Case II

A boy aged 12 years

Fig. 10-2. (a) The brow is prominent and the mandible is small. (b) Marked dorsal scoliosis is evident. (c) The terminal phalanges of the thumb are broad

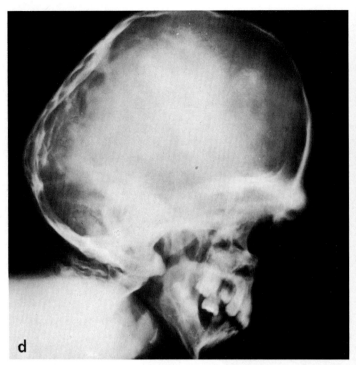

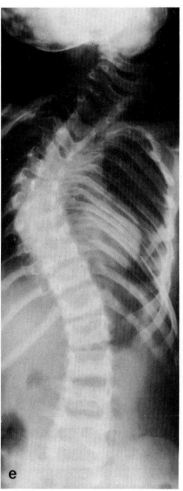

Fig. 10-2. (d) Skull. There is moderate sclerosis of the base and prominence of the supra-orbital ridge. This patient has the characteristic micrognathia together with brachycephaly, not a usual feature (Sellars and Beighton 1978). (e) Spine. There is severe scoliosis and some ribs are attenuated posteriorly

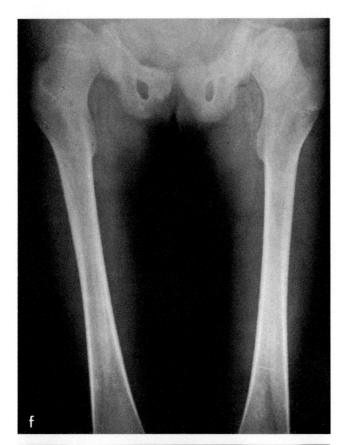

Fig. 10-2. (f) Pelvis and upper femora. Coxa vara and medial deviation of the subtrochanteric portions of the femora are evident

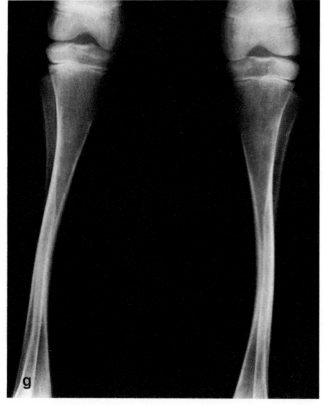

Fig. 10-2. (g) Legs. The tibia have an S-shaped configuration (Sellars and Beighton 1978)

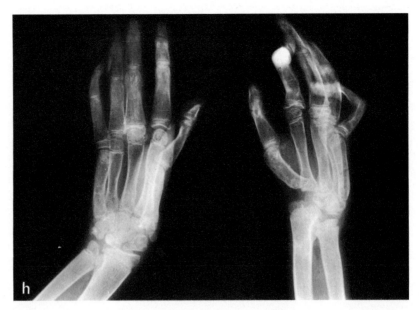

Fig. 10-2. (h) Hands. Modelling of the tubular bones is defective and the proximal phalanges are disproportionately long (Sellars and Beighton 1978)

Chapter 11

Dysosteosclerosis

Historical and Nosological Considerations

SPRANGER et al. (1968) applied the designation 'dysosteosclerosis' to a condition in which short stature and bone fragility are associated with sclerosis of the axial skeleton, platyspondyly, and metaphyseal widening. These authors recognised several similar cases in the literature and other reports have followed. A total of 12 patients have been described, of whom 11 have been males, the eldest being 15 years of age. Details are given in Table 11-1.

Clinical Features

Limb length is short relative to the trunk, and affected individuals are below the normal height for their age. The thorax is constricted with pectus carinatum and a Harrison's sulcus. The face and nose are narrow, the man-

Table 11-1. Dysosteosclerosis – reported cases

Author	Initial diagnosis	Patients	Consanguinity	Country of origin
ELLIS (1934)	Osteopetrosis	Brothers aged $1^1/_2$ and $2^1/_2$	+	Britain
FIELD (1938)	Ellis' patients restudied			
STEHR (1941)	Osteosclerosis	Brothers, 8 and 12		Germany
ROY et al. (1968)	"New syndrome"	Girl, 13		France
SPRANGER et al. (1968)	Dysosteosclerosis	Boy, 10	+	Germany
LEISTI et al. (1975)	Dysosteosclerosis	Boy, 6		U.S.A.
KAITILA and RIMOIN (1976)	Further details of above patient			
PASCUAL-CASTROVIEJO et al. (1977)	X-linked Dysosteosclerosis	4 male cousins in 3 branches of a kindred		Spain
HOUSTON et al. (1978)	Dysosteosclerosis	Boy, 15	+	U.S.A. (German-Mennonite)

dible is small, and the forehead and parietal regions are bulky. Dental development is faulty, with maleruption and caries of the permanent teeth. The bones are fragile and fractures are frequent.

Bony encroachment narrows the foramina of the optic nerves and blindness in infancy is a consistent feature. Several reported patients have been mentally retarded. Progressive bulbar palsy and macular skin atrophy were additional features in a 13-year-old girl described by Roy et al. (1968).

Dysosteosclerosis is apparently a progressive condition but as all reported patients have been children, the long-term course and the ultimate prognosis are unknown.

Radiographic Manifestations

The most prominent diagnostic features in the fully developed cases are sclerosis, platyspondyly and metaphyseal flaring. Houston et al. (1978) depicted the development of radiographic changes in an affected boy from the age of 20 months to 15 years. These authors pointed out that early radiographic changes were reminiscent of osteopetrosis, while in later childhood they resembled craniometaphyseal dysplasia.

Skull

Changes are evident in the skull during infancy. These include sclerosis of the base, mastoid, and paranasal sinuses, with narrowing of the optic nerve canals. The frontal and parietal regions of the calvarium are bulky and closure of the fontanelles may be delayed. There is little or no calvarial hyperostosis and sclerosis of the vault is patchy and much milder than in the base.

Spine

The vertebral bodies become flattened and show dorsal wedging, anterior concavity and irregular sclerosis.

Chest and Pelvis

The ribs are short and sclerotic but may have a triangular radiolucency at their paravertebral ends. The scapulae are dense and the medial portions of the clavicles are expanded.

In infancy, increased density is evident around the margins of the iliac crests. By late childhood, some sclerosis may be apparent in the lower region of each ilium.

Limbs

In infancy, the metaphyses of the long bones are expanded and contain dense transverse bands, while the epiphyses are sclerotic. In later childhood, the ends of these bones are undermodelled and radiolucent, with thin cortices and a few residual patches of sclerosis. These changes are marked in the distal femora, which take on the classical Erlenmeyer flask appearance. By contrast, the mid-diaphyseal portions of the long bones become constricted and their cortices develop endosteal hyperostosis.

The short tubular bones of the extremities show sclerosis of the metaphyses and epiphyses, with diaphyseal lucency. The metacarpals and metatarsals have dense accessory ossification centres, while the small bones of the tarsus and carpus are sclerotic. Bone age is retarded.

Comment

The combination of precocious optic nerve compression, shortness of stature, lack of significant hyperostosis of the calvarium and mandible, and sclerosis and flattening of the vertebral bodies serves to distinguish dysosteosclerosis from other bone dysplasias.

The presence of two sets of affected siblings with normal parents and consanguinity in three reported kindreds is suggestive of autosomal recessive inheritance. However, the presence of the condition in four male cousins with three normal mothers and an unaffected maternal grandmother is strong evidence for X-linked inheritance (PASCUAL-CASTROVIEJO et al. 1977). The fact that 11 of the 12 reported patients have been males supports this contention. As the only reported female (ROY et al. 1968) was somewhat atypical in her neurological and dermatological manifestations, it is possible that dysosteosclerosis is genetically heterogeneous.

References

ELLIS RWB (1934) Osteopetrosis. Proc R Soc Med 27:1563

FIELD CE (1938) Albers-Schönberg disease. An atypical case. Proc R Soc Med 32:320

HOUSTON CS, GERRARD JW, IVES EJ (1978) Dysosteosclerosis A J R 130:988

KAITILA I, RIMOIN DL (1976) Histologic heterogeneity in the hyperostotic bone dysplasias. Birth Defects 12/6:71

LEISTI J, KAITILA I, LACHMAN RS, ASCH MJ, RIMOIN DL (1975) Dysosteosclerosis (Case report). Birth Defects 11/6:349

PASCUAL-CASTROVIEJO I, CASAS-FERNANDEZ C, LOPEZ-MARTIN V, MARTINEZ-BERMEIO A (1977) X-linked dysosteosclerosis. Four familial cases. Eur J Pediatr 126:127

ROY C, MAROTEAUX P, KREMP L, COURTECUISSE V, ALAGILLE D (1968) Un nouveau syndrome osseux avec anomalies cutanées et troubles neurologiques. Arch Fr Pediatr 25:983

SPRANGER J. ALBRECHT C, ROHWEDDER H-J, WIEDEMANN H-R (1968) Die Dysosteosklerose: eine Sonderform der generalisierten Osteosklerose. Fortschr Roentgenstr 109:504

STEHR L (1941) Pathogenese und Klinik der Osteosklerosen. Arch Orthop Unfallchir 41:156

This case is presented by kind permission of Dr. C.S. Houston of the University of Saskatchewan. The patient, now 18 years of age, has severe retardation of maturation and is attending a school for the blind (Houston et al. 1978)

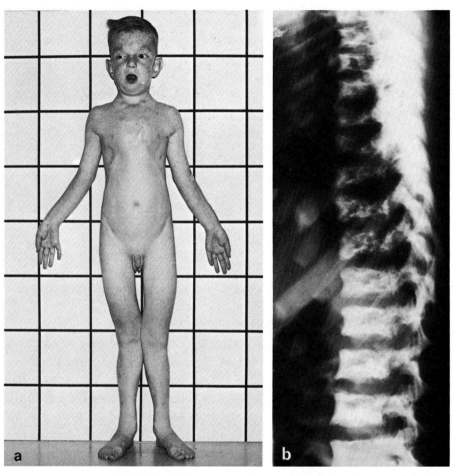

Fig. 11-1. (a) The clinical appearance in early childhood. The nose and midface are narrow and the mandible is small. Thoracic deformity, femoral bowing, and genu valgus are evident

Fig. 11-1. (b) Spine at 15 years. The vertebrae show generalised platyspondyly, irregularity and sclerosis, with anterior concavity

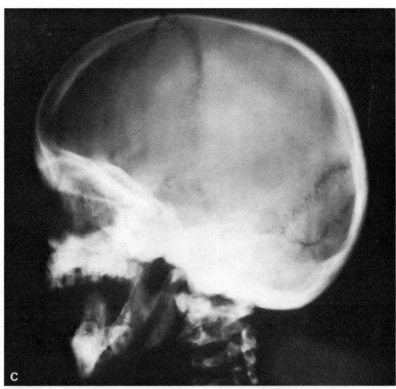

Fig. 11-1. (c) Skull at 5$^1/_2$ years. The base is dense, the mastoids are sclerotic and the paranasal sinuses are not pneumatised

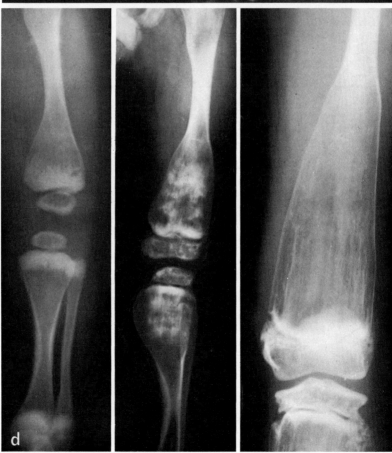

Fig. 11-1. (d) Lower limb at 20 months, 5 years, and 15 years. The radiograph obtained at 20 months demonstrates wide metaphyses with dense bands. At 5 years irregular densities and lack of modelling are evident. At 15 years the distal femur has an Erlenmeyer flask configuration, with cortical thinning and vertical striations

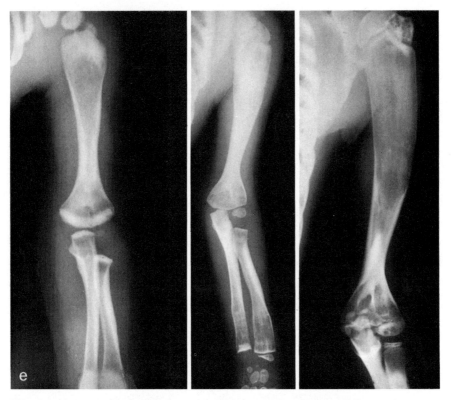

Fig. 11-1. (e) Arm at 20 months, 5 years, and 15 years. The sequence of changes in density pattern and modelling resembles that seen in the lower limbs

Chapter 12

Endosteal Hyperostosis

Historical and Nosological Considerations

The nosology of this condition is confusing, and the designations 'van Buchem disease' and 'hyperostosis corticalis' are better known than the term
'endosteal hyperostosis (van Buchem and other forms)' which was used in
the 1970 Paris Nomenclature. In the 1977 version of the Nomenclature, the
condition was subdivided into autosomal dominant (Worth) and autosomal recessive (van Buchem) types, as shown below:

Endosteal Hyperostosis

1. Autosomal dominant   Autosomal dominant osteosclerosis
   (Worth)
2. Autosomal recessive   Hyperostosis corticalis generalisata familiaris,
   (van Buchem)   or generalised cortical hyperostosis

It must be emphasised that clinical and radiographic differentiation of
these two genetic conditions may be impossible; for this reason they are
considered together in this chapter.

The situation evolved in the following way. The disorder first attracted attention when VAN BUCHEM et al. (1955) used the term 'hyperostosis corticalis
generalisata familiaris' in a report of a brother and sister in Holland, who
had overgrowth and sclerosis of the skull and the diaphyses of the long
bones. Subsequently, VAN BUCHEM et al. (1962) gave further details of these
two patients, together with five others, and FOSMOE et al. (1968) described
a sporadic case, employing the eponym 'van Buchem's disease.' Eight more
affected individuals in a large, inbred kindred on the island of Urk in the
Netherlands were reported by VAN BUCHEM (1971), and the observations on
the whole series of 15 Dutch patients were presented in a comprehensive
monograph by VAN BUCHEM et al. (1976). Pedigree data were indicative of
autosomal recessive inheritance.

WORTH and WOLLIN (1966) encountered generation-to-generation transmission of hyperostosis corticalis generalisata. MAROTEAUX et al. (1971) recognised that there were distinct autosomal dominant and autosomal recessive forms of the condition, and SPRANGER et al. (1974) used the term 'endosteal hyperostosis' to embrace both types. BEALS (1976) described a kin-

dred in which 14 individuals in four generations had 'endosteal hyperostosis,' and a further family with eight cases in four generations was reported by LAPRESLE et al. (1976). OWEN (1976) restudied a woman in Britain who had been described by DYSON (1972) and found five affected relatives in three generations. Five more cases in two kindreds were encountered by VAYSSAIRAT et al. (1976). In the light of this accumulated evidence, GELMAN (1977) and GORLIN and GLASS (1977) employed the term 'autosomal dominant osteosclerosis' to emphasise that this form of the condition was a separate entity.

EASTMAN and BIXLER (1977) analysed 41 published cases and concluded that in addition to the young woman whom they described only six individuals in four reported kindreds had the classic autosomal recessive van Buchem disease. However, this figure underestimates the actual situation, as VAN BUCHEM's third series of eight patients were excluded from this analysis. EASTMAN and BIXLER (1977) confirmed that inheritance was autosomal dominant in several families and suggested that other patients in the group they had analysed might have had sclerosteosis or craniodiaphyseal dysplasia rather than endosteal hyperostosis.

Clinical Features

Progressive asymmetrical enlargement of the mandible with onset in late childhood is the usual presenting feature, and apart from this problem, affected individuals may remain asymptomatic. Mild prominence of the forehead and widening of the nasal bridge with nasal obstruction may develop, but head circumference is not increased. Facial nerve palsy and deafness are inconsistent complications, but compression of the optic nerves is unusual. In general, cranial nerve complications are much more common in the van Buchem form of the condition (see Table 12-1). Owing to diagnostic uncertainty in some reported cases, the true incidence of these problems has not been established.

The intellect and habitus are normal, general health is good, and the bones are not fragile.

The serum alkaline phosphatase is sometimes raised in the autosomal recessive form but is normal in the autosomal dominant type. Biochemical and haemotological studies yield otherwise normal results.

Radiographic Manifestations

Sclerosis of the skull, enlargement of the jaw, and thickening of the diaphyseal cortices of the long bones are the major features of endosteal hyperostosis. The tubular bones are not undermodelled.

Table 12-1. Possible distinguishing features of autosomal dominant (Worth) and autosomal recessive (VAN BUCHEM) types of endosteal hyperostosis

	AD form (Worth)	AR form (van Buchem)
Periosteal excrescences	Absent	Present
Cranial nerve palsy	Infrequent	Frequent
Severity	Mild	Moderate
Pattern of inheritance	AD	AR

Skull

The calvarium is sclerotic and widened with loss of distinction between the tables. The base of the skull is sclerotic, but the air sinuses are patent. The mandible is markedly hyperostotic and the mandibular angle may be increased.

Spine

Some degree of sclerosis is present in the vertebral bodies, but their external contours are undisturbed.

Chest and Pelvis

The ribs, clavicles, scapulae and pelvis may have a coarse, trabecular pattern or show diffuse sclerosis without significant widening.

Limbs

The diaphyses of the long bones show increased cortical thickness and sclerosis, with diminution of the medullary cavity. The outlines of the bones may be mildly distorted but there are no modelling defects. Similar but mild changes are present in the tubular bones of the extremities.

Periosteal excrescences have been observed on the shafts of the tubular bones in some patients, but these are by no means a consistent feature.

Comment

JACOBS (1977) gave further details of an affected boy previously reported by SCOTT and GAUTBY (1974) and reviewed the clinical, radiographic, genetic, and pathological aspects of the disorder. He pointed out that the dominant form tends to be benign and that overgrowth of the jaw may be the only clinical feature. In contrast, facial deformity is more severe and cranial nerve compression is more frequent in the recessive type.

The severe autosomal recessive form of endosteal hyperostosis resembles sclerosteosis (see Chap. 13). Distinguishing features of this latter entity are gigantism and syndactyly, together with cranial nerve palsies and elevation of intracranial pressure in adulthood.

Craniodiaphyseal dysplasia (see Chap. 11) may also be a source of confusion, but in this condition there is more involvement of the cranium and less cortical thickening in the tubular bones.

References

BEALS RK (1976) Endosteal hyperostosis. J Bone Joint Surg [Am] 58:1172

DYSON DP (1972) Van Buchem's disease (Hyperostosis corticalis generalisata familiaris). Br J Oral S 9:237

EASTMAN JR, BIXLER D (1977) Generalised cortical hyperostosis (Van Buchem disease): Nosologic considerations. Radiology 125:297

FOSMOE RJ, HOLM RS, HILDRETH RC (1968) Van Buchem's Disease (Hyperostosis corticalis generalisata familiaris). A case report. Radiology 90:771

GELMAN MI (1977) Autosomal dominant osteosclerosis. Radiology 125:289

GORLIN RJ, GLASS L (1977) Autosomal dominant osteosclerosis. Radiology 125:547

JACOBS P (1977) Van Buchem disease. Postgrad Med J 53:497

LAPRESLE J, MAROTEAUX P, KUFFER R, SAID G, MEYER O (1976) Hyperostose corticale généralisée dominante avec atteinte multiple des nerfs crânies. Nouv Presse Méd 5/40:2703

MAROTEAUX P, FONTAINE G, SCHARFMAN W, FARRIAUX JP (1971) L'hyperostose corticale généralisée à transmission dominante. Arch Fr Pédiatr 28:685

OWEN RH (1976) Van Buchem's disease. Br J Radiol 49:126

RUSSELL WJ, BIZZOZERO OJ, OMORI Y (1968) Idiopathic osteosclerosis. A report of 6 related cases. Radiology 90:70

SCOTT WC, GAUTBY THT (1974) Hyperostosis corticalis generalisata familiaris. Br J Radiol 47:500

SPRANGER JW, LANGER LO, WIEDEMANN HR (1974) Bone dysplasias. An atlas of constitutional disorders of skeletal development. Saunders, Philadelphia, p 331

VAN BUCHEM FSP (1971) Hyperostosis corticalis generalisata. Eight new cases. Acta Med Scand 189:257

VAN BUCHEM FSP, HADDERS HN, UBBENS R (1955) An uncommon familial systemic disease of the skeleton. Hyperostosis corticalis generalisata familiaris. Acta Radiol (Stockh) 44:109

VAN BUCHEM FSP, HADDERS HN, HANSEN JF, WOLDRING MG (1962) Hyperostosis corticalis generalisata. Report of seven cases. Am J Med 33:387

VAN BUCHEM FSP, PRICK JJG, JASPAR HHJ (1976) Hyperostosis corticalis generalisata familiaris (Van Buchem's disease). American Elsevier, New York

VAYSSAIRAT M, PRIER A, MEISEL C (1976) New cases of familial generalized cortical hyperostosis with dominant transmission (Worth's type). J Radiol Electrol Méd Nucl 57/10:719

WORTH HM, WOLLIN DG (1966) Hyperostosis corticalis generalisata congenita. J Can Assoc Radiol. 17:67

These cases of the Worth, or autosomal dominant, form of endosteal hyperostosis are presented by kind permission of Dr R.H. Owen of Chepstow and Dr W.C. Scott of Dorset, U.K.

Case I
Female, aged 40 years (Owen 1976)

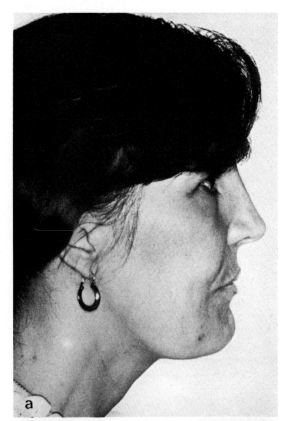

Fig. 12-1. (a) Profile. The mandible is prominent but the face is otherwise normal.

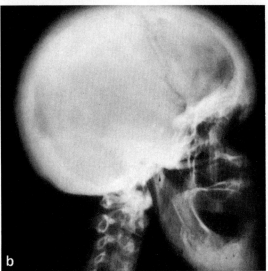

Fig. 12-1. (b) Skull. The mandible and calvarium show marked thickening and increased density

Fig. 12-1. (c) Mandible, oblique view. The
mandible is sclerotic and expanded. (d) Pelvis.
Bone texture is normal, apart from coarse
sclerosis above the acetabula. (e) Arm.
Endosteal cortical thickening is present in the
shaft of the humerus

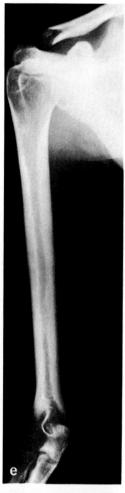

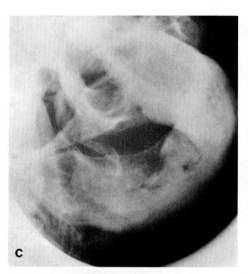

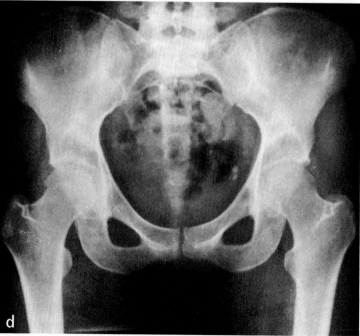

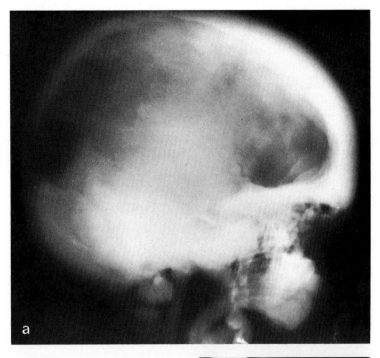

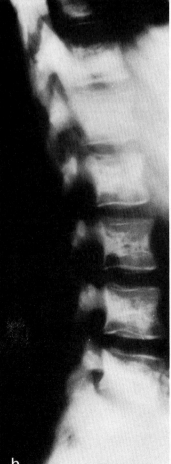

Case II
Male, aged 17 years (Scott and Gautby 1974)

Fig. 12-2. (a) Skull. Marked sclerosis is present in the vault, base and maxilla. (b) Spine. Unusual horizontal striations are evident

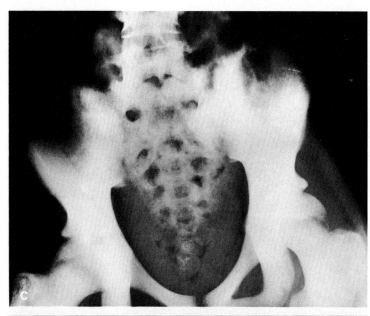

Fig. 12-2. (c) Pelvis. Generalised sclerosis

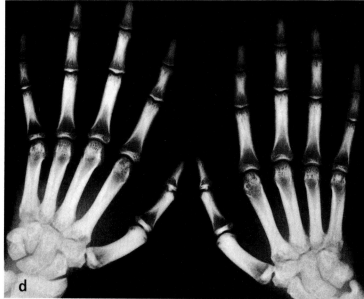

Fig. 12-2. (d) Hands. The cortices of the metacarpals and phalanges are widened and sclerotic but the external bony contours are undisturbed

Chapter 13

Sclerosteosis

Historical and Nosological Considerations

Sclerosteosis was first recognised as a distinct entity when TRUSWELL (1958) described two unrelated South African girls with 'osteopetrosis with syndactyly; a morphological variant of Albers-Schönberg disease.' Subsequently, HANSEN (1967) used the term 'sklerosteose,' which in its anglicised form 'sclerosteosis' has gained general acceptance.

A retrospective diagnosis of sclerosteosis can be made in the South African patients reported by FALCONER and RYRIE (1937) and KLINTWORTH (1963). The only reports from outside South Africa have concerned a set of siblings in New York (HIGINBOTHAM and ALEXANDER 1941), a young woman in Switzerland (PIETRUSCHKA 1958), and a girl in Japan (SUGIURA and YASUHARA 1975). A Negro kindred in the United States of America in which four siblings had 'Albers-Schönberg disease,' reported by KELLEY and LAWLAH (1946) and later cited by WITKOP (1965), has also been quoted as an example of sclerosteosis.

The manifestations in 25 affected Afrikaners were reviewed by BEIGHTON et al. (1976), and a further 17 patients were reported by BEIGHTON and HAMERSMA (1979).

Clinical Features

Mandibular prognathism and frontal prominence become evident by the age of five years. These deformities progress and in adulthood the face is severely distorted, with dental malocclusion, proptosis and relative mid-facial hypoplasia. Affected children are tall for their age, and adults with the condition may have gigantism. The majority have partial or total syndactyly, usually of the second and third fingers, with deviation of the terminal phalanges and hypoplasia of the nails on the corresponding digits. The bones are resistant to trauma and fractures are infrequent.

Transient palsy of the seventh cranial nerve occurs during infancy, and bilateral facial paralysis is usually permanent by adulthood. Progressive bony encroachment upon the middle ear cavities and auditory nerve canals often causes deafness in mid-childhood. Compression of the optic nerves is a late complication.

Overgrowth of the calvarium leads to progressive diminution of the capacity of the cranial cavity, with elevation of intracranial pressure. Severe headache due to this mechanism often develops in early adulthood and several patients have died suddenly from impaction of the medulla oblongata in the foramen magnum. Prophylactic craniotomy should be considered in all adult patients.

Radiographic Manifestations

Some cranial thickening and sclerosis may be evident in infancy and widespread changes are well advanced by the age of five years. Hyperostosis progresses until the end of the third decade, when the condition becomes static. The radiographic manifestations of sclerosteosis have been reviewed by BEIGHTON et al. (1976b).

Skull

The calvarium is widened and uniformly sclerotic. The base becomes very dense and the cranial nerve foramina may be obliterated. The sinuses remain patent and the sella turcica may be expanded. The mandible is dense and massive, with asymmetrical distortion and dental malocclusion.

Spine

The vertebral end plates and pedicles are sclerotic but the outlines of the bodies are not disturbed.

Chest and Pelvis

The clavicles and ribs are widened and dense and the scapulae and pelvis are sclerotic but not expanded.

Limbs

The long bones are massive, with cortical hyperostosis and moderate alteration of their external contours. All the tubular bones, including those of the extremities, are involved in this process. Irregular cortical thickening is a mild but variable feature and is apparently age-related.

Syndactyly, which is most often present in the second and third fingers, ranges from complete bony union to minimal skin webbing. Radial deviation of the terminal phalanges may be radiologically evident. The toes are not syndactylous.

Table 13-1. Distinguishing features of Sclerosteosis and van Buchem disease

	Sclerosteosis	van Buchem disease
Reported cases	50	15
Age of clinical presentation	Early childhood	Puberty
Prognosis	Potentially lethal	Benign
Habitus	Gigantism	Normal stature
Facies	Gross distortion	Prominent mandible
Cranial nerve palsy	Very common	Inconsistent
Intracranial pressure	Elevated	Normal
Syndactyly	Frequent	Absent
Nail hypoplasia	Frequent	Absent
Cranial hyperostosis	Gross	Moderate
Distortion of tubular bones of hands and feet	Marked	Mild

Comment

Sclerosteosis is very similar to the autosomal recessive form of endosteal hyperostosis (van Buchem disease, see Chap. 12), and as many of the Afrikaners of South Africa had their origins in Holland, where VAN BUCHEM's patients were studied, it seems possible that there might be some fundamental link between these disorders. They are both inherited as autosomal recessives and the clinical and radiographic manifestations are similar. Distinguishing features are shown in Table 13-1.

Both sclerosteosis and van Buchem disease are progressive and Table 13-1 pertains to the situation in the affected adult in whom the manifestations are fully developed. No absolute diagnostic marker has yet been recognised (EPSTEIN et al. 1979), and changes such as periosteal excrescences or elevated levels of serum alkaline phosphatase, which have been discussed in this context, are unhelpful, as they may occur in both conditions.

In view of the high prevalence of sclerosteosis in the Afrikaner population of South Africa, the condition should be suspected in any member of this community who presents with syndactyly or facial palsy. As cranial sclerosis is evident in infancy, the diagnosis can be confirmed radiologically at an early stage. Antenatal diagnosis has not yet been achieved, but in the future it might be possible to recognise syndactyly in a potentially affected fetus by means of sophisticated fetoscopic techniques. Similarly, the presence of minor radiographic changes in the skulls of heterozygous carriers of the gene may eventually prove to be of value in genetic counselling and prevention (BEIGHTON et al. 1977).

References

BEIGHTON P, HAMERSMA H (1979) Sclerosteosis in South Africa. S Afr Med J 55:783

BEIGHTON P, DAVIDSON J, DURR L, HAMERSMA H (1977) Sclerosteosis – An autosomal recessive disorder. Clin Genet 11:1

BEIGHTON P, CREMIN BJ, HAMERSMA H (1976a) The radiology of sclerosteosis. Brit J Radiol 49:934

BEIGHTON P, DURR L, HAMERSMA H (1976b) The clinical features of sclerosteosis. A review of the manifestations in twenty-five affected individuals. Ann Intern Med 84:393

CREMIN BJ (1979) Sclerosteosis in children. Pediatr Radiol 8:173

EPSTEIN S, HAMERSMA H, BEIGHTON P (1979) Endocrine function in sclerosteosis. S Afr Med 55:1105

FALCONER AW, RYRIE BJ (1937) Report on a familial type of generalised osteosclerosis. Med Press 195:12

HANSEN HG (1967) Sklerosteose. In: OPITZ H, SCHMIDT F (eds) Handbuch der Kinderheilkunde, vol 6, Springer, Berlin Heidelberg New York, p 351

HIGINBOTHAM NL, ALEXANDER SF (1941) Osteopetrosis. Four cases in one family. Am J Surg 53:444

KELLEY CH, LAWLAH JW (1946) Albers-Schönberg disease – A family survey. Radiology 47:507

KLINTWORTH GK (1963) The neurologic manifestations of osteopetrosis (Albers-Schönberg's disease) Neurology (Minneap) 13:512

SUGIURA Y, YASUHARA T (1975) Sclerosteosis. A case report. J Bone Joint Surg [Am] 57:273

PIETRUSCHKA G (1958) Weitere Mitteilungen über die Marmorknochenkrankheit (Albers-Schönbergsche Krankheit) nebst Bemerkungen zur Differentialdiagnose. Klin Monatsbl Augenheilk 132:509

TRUSWELL AS (1958) Osteopetrosis with syndactyly. A morphological variant of Albers-Schönberg disease. J Bone Joint Surg 40:208

WITKOP CJ (1965) Genetic disease of the oral cavity. In: TIECKE RW (ed) Oral Pathology. McGraw-Hill, New York

Sclerosis and hyperostosis of the cranium and cortices of the tubular bones become evident in infancy and progress throughout the period of growth. Two cases are presented to demonstrate the age relationship of these changes. Case 1 is a girl whom we have studied from the age of 10 to 16 years. Case 2 is a male aged 44 years who shows the fully developed radiological manifestations. Finally, montages of skulls and hands of different patients are shown to illustrate the spectrum of changes in these areas

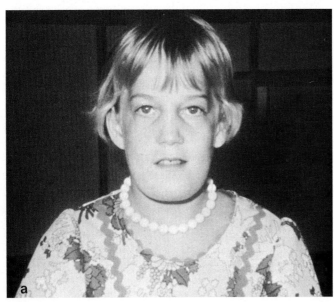

Case I

Fig. 13-1. (a) Girl aged 10 years, with a prominent and bulky mandible. Bone overgrowth has already caused deafness and facial palsy (Beighton and Hamersma 1979)

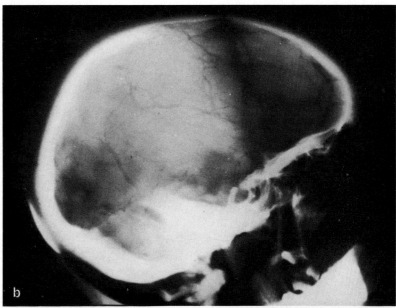

Fig. 13-1. (b) Skull. Lateral view at 10 years, showing sclerosis which is most marked in the base and occipital regions

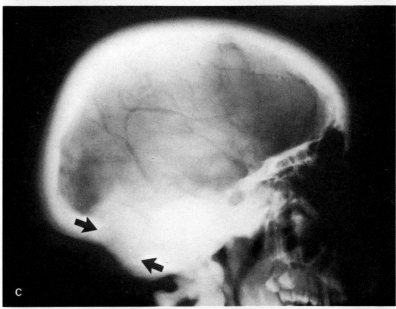

Fig. 13-1. (c) Skull. Lateral view at 16 years demonstrating progression of sclerosis of the calvarium and base. Arrows indicate a recent craniotomy site (see also Fig. 13-1)

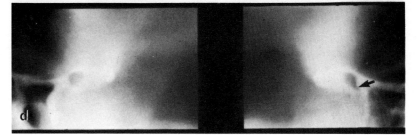

Fig. 13-1. (d) Optic formina shown by multidirectional tomography. There is slight narrowing of the left optic foramen (arrow)

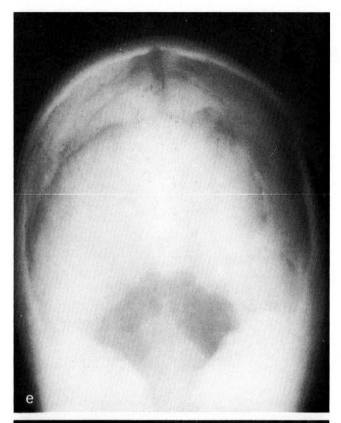

Fig. 13-1. (e) Townes view, showing extreme density of the petrous bones and base of the skull. The foramen magnum has been surgically enlarged

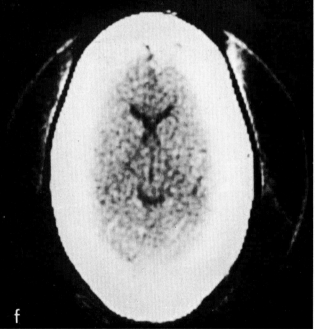

Fig. 13-1. (f) C.T. Scan at 2A level. Calvarial thickening is gross but the ventricles are normal in size (Cremin 1979)

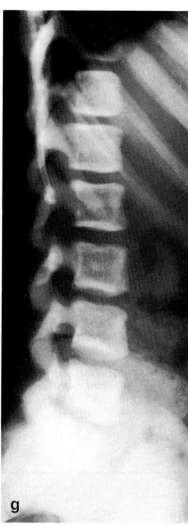

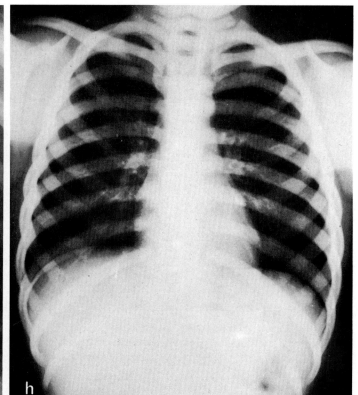

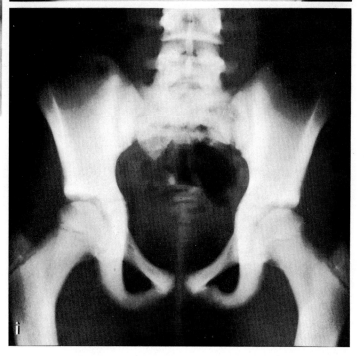

Fig. 13-1. (g) Spine. Lateral view showing a mild degree of increased density of the posterior elements and end plates of the bodies. (h) Chest. The ribs and clavicles show moderate cortical sclerosis and hyperostosis. (i) Pelvis. Sclerosis is generalised but the bone contours are undisturbed

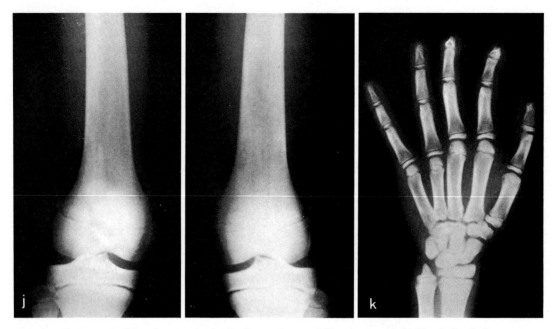

Fig. 13-1. (j) Knees. A diffuse increase in density is seen but modelling is normal. (k) Hand. Cortical thickening and faulty modelling of the metacarpals and phalanges is present. Dysplasia and radial deviation of the terminal phalanges of the second and third fingers is a variable feature

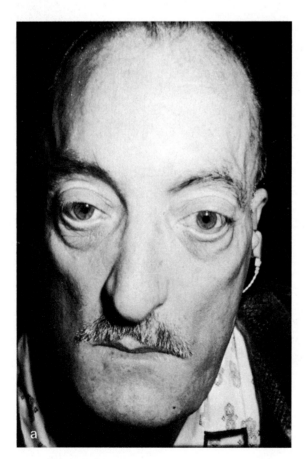

Case II
Male aged 33 years

Fig. 13-2. (a) The mandible is prominent and asymmetrical and there is proptosis and left facial palsy. A hearing aid is worn (Beighton et al. 1976)

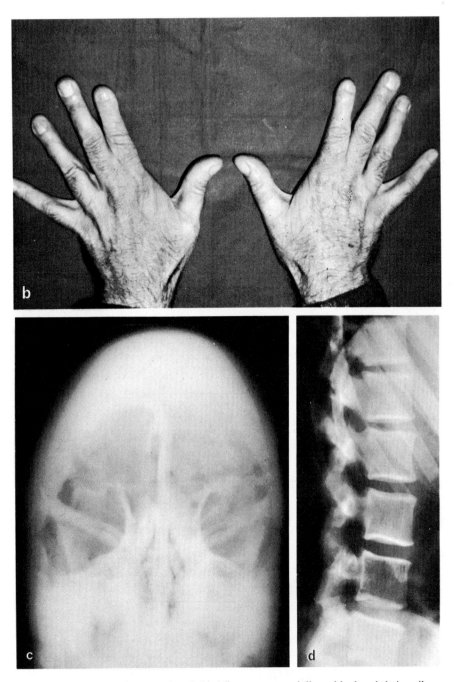

Fig. 13-2. (b) Hands. The second and third fingers are partially webbed and their nails are hypoplastic. (c) Skull. Frontal view demonstrating severe sclerosis of the vault and maxilla. (d) Spine. The vertebral bodies and pedicles are relatively normal (Beighton et al. 1976a, b)

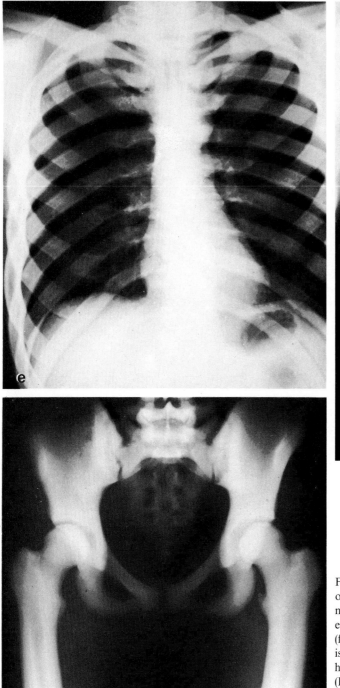

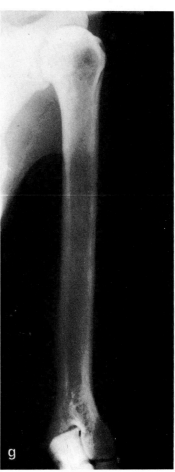

Fig. 13-2. (e) Chest. Mild sclerosis of the ribs and widening of the medial ends of the clavicles are evident (Beighton et al. 1976a). (f) Pelvis. Diffuse uniform sclerosis is present. Cortical sclerosis and hyperostosis are seen in the femora (Beighton et al. 1976a). (g) Arm. Pronounced cortical hyperostosis is present (Beighton et al. 1976a)

Skull Montage

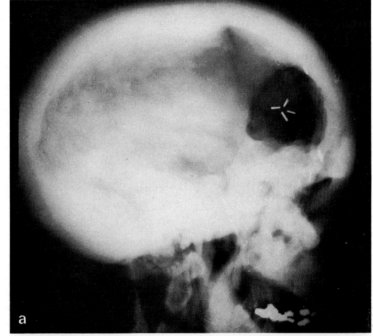

Fig. 13-3. (a) Female aged 23. The calvarium, base and mandible are diffusely sclerotic. Frontal craniotomy has been undertaken to relieve elevated intracranial pressure (Beighton et al. 1976b; Epstein et al. 1979)

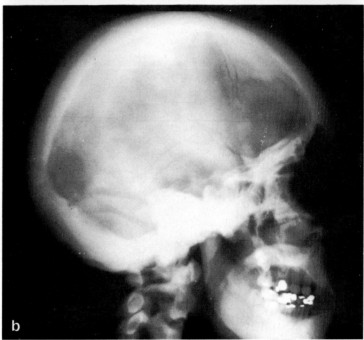

Fig. 13-3. (b) Female aged 25. Marked sclerosis, with loss of distinction between the tables of the vault. Involvement of the mandible is severe (Beighton et al. 1977)

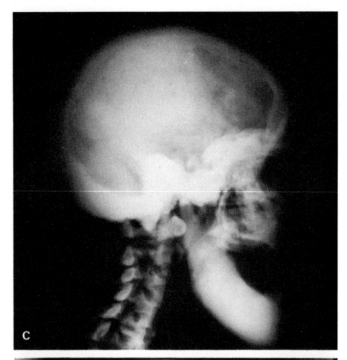

Fig. 13-3. (c) Male aged 32. The base is very sclerotic. Hyperostosis and sclerosis of the mandible is unusually severe

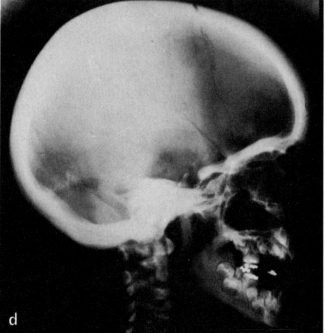

Fig. 13-3. (d) Female aged 36. Moderate sclerosis and thickening of the skull base and calvarium are evident but the mandible is relatively spared

Hand Montage

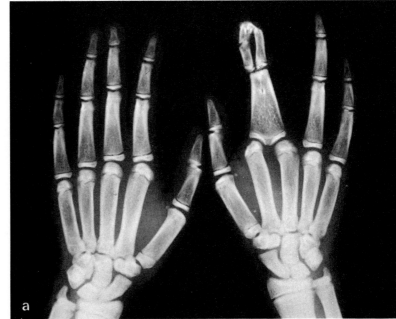

Fig. 13-4. (a) Boy aged 16. The metacarpals and phalanges show defective modelling. Bony syndactyly is present, involving the left index and middle fingers (Beighton and Hamersma 1979)

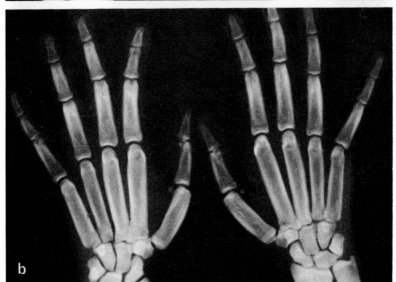

Fig. 13-4. (b) Female aged 23 years. The metacarpals and phalanges show marked undermodelling and moderate cortical hyperostosis

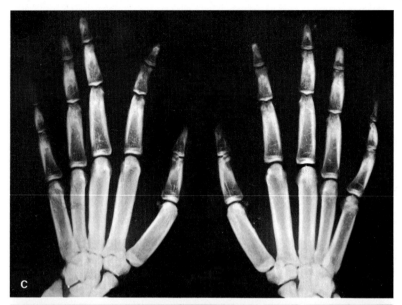

Fig. 13-4. (c) Female aged 23 years. Soft-tissue syndactyly, of varying degree has been corrected in these patients. (Beighton and Hamersma 1979)

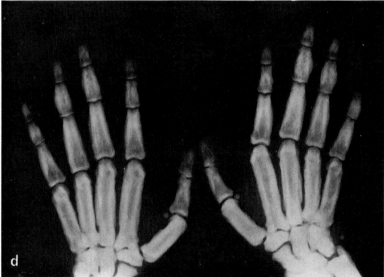

Fig. 13-4. (d) Male aged 55 years. The tubular bones show massive cortical overgrowth and sclerosis and their external contours are very irregular (Beighton and Hamersma 1979)

Chapter 14

Diaphyseal Dysplasia (Camurati-Engelmann Disease)

Historical and Nosological Consideration

CAMURATI (1922) described a seven-year-old boy with painful lower limbs and diaphyseal cortical thickening in the long bones of the legs. The 55-year-old father and eight of their family members in four generations were thought to be affected, and the condition was termed 'hereditary symmetrical osteitis'.

ENGELMANN (1929) reported an eight-year-old boy with similar clinical and radiographic changes, together with muscle wasting and sclerosis of the skull, under the designation 'osteopathia hyperostotica (sclerotisans) multiplex infantalis.'

The condition received eponymous recognition when SEAR (1948) employed the term 'Engelmann's disease.' Concurrently, NEUHAUSER et al. (1948) used the descriptive designation 'progressive diaphyseal dysplasia.' Subsequently, the conjoined eponym 'Camurati-Engelmann disease' has been used by some authors; others have preferred 'diaphyseal dysplasia.' More than 100 patients have now been reported.

Hereditary multiple diaphyseal sclerosis, described by RIBBING (1949) and PAUL (1953), is almost certainly the same condition as Camurati-Engelmann disease.

Clinical Features

In the classical case, leg pains, muscle weakness and disturbance in gait develop during childhood. Muscle mass is diminished but bony thickening in the lower legs produces a tubular configuration below the knees. Delayed sexual maturation is sometimes a feature and a minority of the affected individuals develop blindness, deafness or facial palsy, due to cranial nerve compression. General health remains good and symptoms often remit in adulthood. There is a wide variation in severity, even within the same kindred, and the manifestations of the disease range from minor symptoms to severe physical handicap. Mildly affected persons may remain totally asymptomatic.

The orthopaedic problems in diaphyseal dysplasia have been reviewed by GRIFFITHS (1956) and CLAWSON and LOOP (1964); the place for corticosteriod treatment has been discussed by ALLEN et al. (1970). YEN et al. (1978) pointed out that optic nerve decompression does not necessarily convey lasting benefit, as bony encroachment in the optic canals may redevelop.

Radiographic Manifestations

As with the clinical features, the radiographic manifestations are age-related and variable in severity. NEUHAUSER et al. (1948) listed the criteria for radiographic diagnosis, and these were used by ANDERSON (1953) and SINGLETON et al. (1956) as a basis for their case reports. Little of note has been added, and the criteria were unchanged when GIRDANY et al. (1973) reviewed the radiographic features of the condition. The scintigraphic appearances of the affected bones have been depicted by STY et al. (1978).

Skull

Changes in the skull are not a prominent feature, although many patients have some degree of cranial sclerosis. This is generally mild and is most often seen in the base, involving the anterior and middle fossa. In more severe cases, the mandible, facial bones and calvarium are also affected.

Spine

Involvement of the spine is unusual but the vertebral bodies and pedicles may be sclerotic, especially in the cervical region.

Chest and Pelvis

The chest and pelvis are usually normal.

Limbs

The long bones of the limbs show symmetrical fusiform expansion of the diaphyses, and the femora and tibiae are always involved. New bone forms on the periosteal and endosteal surfaces of the cortices, and normal trabeculation is lost in the affected areas. The lesion is limited to the diaphyses and has an abrupt demarcation. The epiphyses and metaphyses of the long bones are normal and the short tubular bones of the hands and feet are not affected.

Table 14-1. Diaphyseal dysplasia and craniodiaphyseal dysplasia; distinguishing features

	Diaphyseal dysplasia	Craniodiaphyseal dysplasia
Reported cases	100+	10
Inheritance	Autosomal dominant	Autosomal recessive
Clinical features		
Facial distortion	−	+++
Cranial nerve palsy	+−	++
Muscular involvement	+	−
Progression	−	+
Remission	+	−
Radiographic features		
Cranial sclerosis	+	+++
Diaphyseal expansion	+	+
Metaphyseal involvement	−	+−

Comment

Diaphyseal dysplasia is a reasonably well-defined entity, although patients with severe skull involvement may be difficult to distinguish from individuals with a mild form of craniodiaphyseal dysplasia (see Chap. 8). In general, however, the different clinical courses and genetic backgrounds of these two conditions permit differentiation. Diagnostic features are shown in Table 14-1.

In a review of the clinical and genetic features, SPARKES and GRAHAM (1972) were able to identify 33 sporadic individuals, together with 31 males and 30 females in 20 kindreds. Autosomal dominant inheritance is well established, but non-penetrance is not unusual. In a report of seven cases in three generations of a North American kindred, HUNDLEY and WILSON (1973) emphasised that phenotypic expression was very variable. It is also possible that diaphyseal dysplasia is heterogeneous.

There is no unitary hypothesis to explain the interrelationship of the skeletal and muscular changes in diaphyseal dysplasia. The course of the condition, with stasis or resolution at adulthood, is unusual, and detailed studies of calcium and phosphorous metabolism have failed to elucidate the pathogenesis (SMITH et al. 1977).

References

ALLEN DT, SAUNDERS AM, NORTHWAY WH JR, WILLIAMS GF, SCHAFER IA (1970) Corticosteroids in the treatment of Engelmann's disease: Progressive diaphyseal dysplasia. Pediatrics 46:523

ANDERSON FG (1953) Engelmann's disease. Br J Radiol 26:603

CAMURATI M (1922) Di un raro caso di osteite simmetrica ereditaria degli arti inferiori. Chir Organi Mov 6:662

CLAWSON DK, LOOP JW (1964) Progressive diaphyseal dysplasia (Engelmann's disease). J Bone Joint Surg [Am] 46:143

ENGELMANN G (1929) Ein Fall von Osteopathia Hyperostica (sclerotisans) Multiplex Infantalis. Fortschr Roentgenstr 39:1101

GIRDANY BR, SANE S, GRAHAM CB (1973) Engelmann's disease. In: KAUFMANN HJ (ed) Intrinsic diseases of bones. Basel, Karger (Progress in pediatric radiology, vol 4, p 414)

GRIFFITHS DL (1956) Engelmann's disease. J Bone Joint Surg 38:312

HUNDLEY JD, WILSON FC (1973) Progressive diaphyseal dysplasia. J Bone Joint Surg [Am] 55:461

NEUHAUSER EB, SCHWACHMAN H, WITTENBORG M, COHEN J (1948) Progressive diaphyseal dysplasia. Radiology 51:11

PAUL LW (1953) Hereditary multiple diaphyseal sclerosis (Ribbing). Radiology 60:412

RIBBING S (1949) Hereditary multiple diaphyseal sclerosis. Acta Radiol (Stockh) 31:522

SEAR HR (1948) Engelmann's disease: Osteopathia hyperostotica sclerotisans multiplex infantilis. Report of a case. Br J Radiol 21:236

SINGLETON EB, THOMAS JR, WORTHINGTON WW, HILD JR (1956) Progressive diaphyseal dysplasia (Engelmann's disease). Radiology 67:233

SMITH R, WALTON RJ, CORNER BD, GORDON IRS (1977) Clinical and biochemical studies in Engelmann's disease (Progressive diaphyseal dysplasia). Q J Med 46:273

SPARKES RS, GRAHAM CB (1972) Camurati-Engelmann disease. Genetics and clinical manifestations. J Med Genet 9:73

STY JR, BABBITT DP, STARSHAK RJ (1978) Bone scintigraphy demonstrating Engelmann's disease. Clin Nucl Med 3:69

YEN JK, BOURKE RS, POPP AJ, WIRTH CR (1978) Camurati-Engelmann disease (Progressive hereditary craniodiaphyseal dysplasia): case report. J Neurosurg 48:138

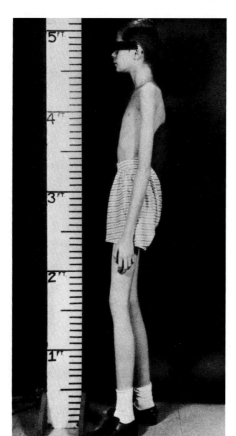

Three cases are presented. The first by courtesy of Dr B.R. Girdany, Children's Hospital, Pittsburgh, and the second by courtesy of Dr I.M. Patz, Middelburg, Transvaal, South Africa

Case I

Boy aged 12 years (Girdany et al. 1973)

Fig. 14-1. This patient has the typical thin habitus

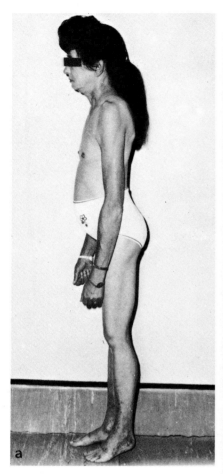

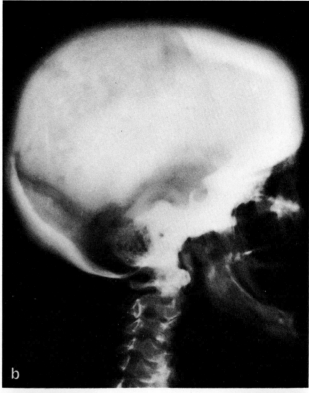

Case II

This patient was first reported by
Dr. Patz in the *South African Medical
Journal* 36, 116–119, 1960. The following
radiographs taken in 1978 showed that
the sclerosis had progressed in skull
and long bones

Fig. 14-2. (a) The resemblance to the
previous case was more marked in the
original publication. (b) Skull.
Hyperostosis involving the vault and
base. Sclerosis is present in over
50 per cent of reported cases, but
changes of this degree are unusual.
(c) Thoracic inlet showing sclerosis of
the medial ends of the clavicles

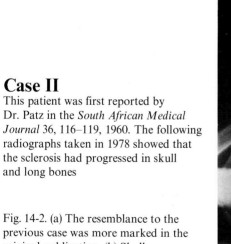

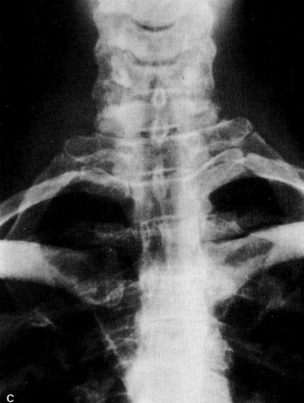

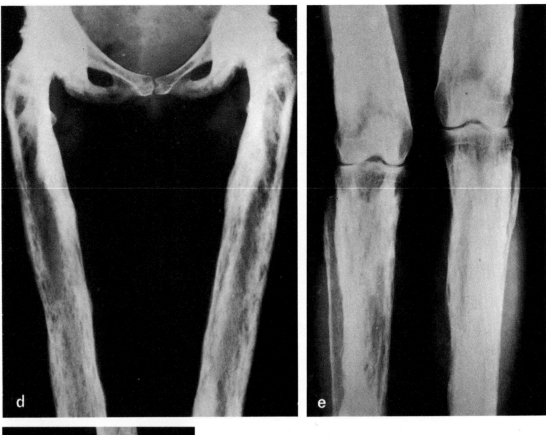

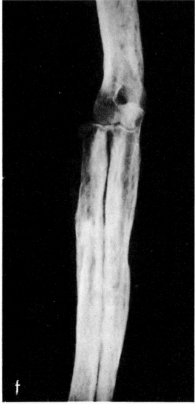

Fig. 14-2. (d–f) Radiographs of proximal femora, distal femora and proximal tibiae, distal humerus and proximal radius and ulna. Internal and external hyperostosis is present to such a degree that Paget disease is simulated. Irregular 'excrescences' are present in the tibae. The hyperostosis predominantly involves the shafts but the metaphyses show some slight encroachment

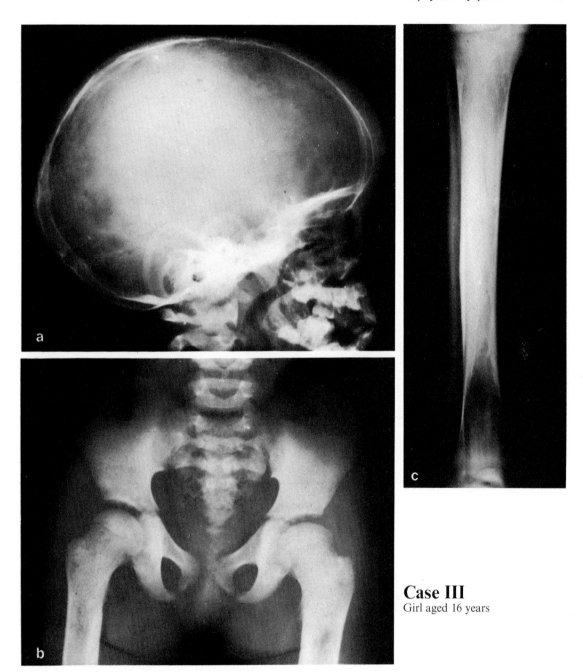

Case III
Girl aged 16 years

Fig. 14-3. (a) Skull. The appearance of the skull in this patient was normal.
(b) Pelvis. Cortical hyperostosis is evident in the proximal femoral shafts.
(c) Leg. The midshaft region of the tibia shows marked sclerosis and thickening

Chapter 15

Osteopathia Striata

Historical and Nosological Considerations

VOORHOEVE (1924) observed linear striations in the long bones and pelvis of a father and his son and daughter, and FAIRBANK (1925) reported another similar case, employing the term 'osteopathia striata' to describe the radiological changes. The condition was initially accepted as a clinically unimportant variant, and this concept still held true when FAIRBANK (1950) reviewed his material 25 years later. Subsequently, the association between bony striations and cranial sclerosis was noted and it was recognised that deafness or minor spinal problems could be inconsistent components of this syndrome (HURT 1953; BLOOR 1954; RUCKER and ALFIDI 1964; JONES and MULCAHY 1968; TAYBI and NUROCK 1969; WALKER 1969; DE BOER and VAN GOOL 1974; FRANKLYN and WILKINSON 1978). The autosomal dominant inheritance of the osteopathia striata–cranial sclerosis syndrome was established by HORAN and BEIGHTON (1978), following a review of four families with the disorder.

Bone striations, in the absence of cranial sclerosis, can occur sporadically and they are also a feature of a number of well-defined syndromes, including osteopetrosis, osteopoikilosis, melorheostosis and focal dermal hypoplasia (LARRÉGUE et al. 1972). In the neonate, a transient 'celery stick' appearance, which is seen in rubella embryopathy and some cases of congenital syphylis, probably represents a similar disturbance in the growth pattern. It must be emphasised that the term 'osteopathia striata' is also used in the non-specific descriptive sense for the radiological appearance of linear skeletal striations, irrespective of their syndromic associations. The osteopathia striata–cranial sclerosis syndrome forms the subject of this chapter, and mention is also made of focal dermal hypoplasia.

Clinical Features

Clinical expression of the osteopathia striata–cranial sclerosis gene is variable, and affected individuals may be totally asymptomatic. Increased head circumference, frontal bossing, and deafness are the most common presenting features. Hearing impairment may result from meatal atresia, middle-

or inner-ear involvement, or bony compression of the auditory nerve. Pectus excavatum, spinal malalignment, and lumbosacral spondylosis are occasionally present.

Height, habitus and intelligence are normal and there are no systemic ramifications.

Radiographic Features

In a number of instances, bony striations and cranial sclerosis have been encountered in the absence of any clinical stigmata and the diagnosis has been made by chance.

Skull

In a typical case, the base of the skull is sclerotic, while the calvarium may be mildly widened and dense. The calvarial changes may be generalised or restricted to the anterior or posterior regions of the skull. The sinuses may be diminished in size or obliterated.

Spine

There are no prominent features but the vertebrae may show mild end-plate sclerosis. Thoracolumbar scoliosis, lumbosacral spondylosis, and deficiency of the pars interarticularis of the vertebral peduncles have been reported.

Chest and Pelvis

Involvement is not marked, but the ribs and pelvis show some patchy sclerosis and fan-shaped linear striations may occur in the ilia.

Limbs

Fine, vertical striations are a characteristic feature in the tubular bones; the sites of predilection are the distal femur, upper tibia and femoral necks. Patchy sclerosis is seen in the carpus and tarsus and in the diaphyses of the long bones.

Comment

Because of the paucity of records and the relatively innocuous nature of the condition, the natural history of the osteopathia striata–cranial sclerosis syndrome has not been comprehensively documented. However, long term follow-up of the female patient of Bloor (1954) and comparison of new radiographs with the originals in the Fairbank collection of the Royal National Orthopaedic Hospital, London showed that there had been little change in the bony appearances in this patient between the ages of 3 and 26 years (HORAN and BEIGHTON 1978).

At the present time about 20 affected individuals in ten kindreds have been reported, but as the gene can be clinically silent, it is likely that the condition is more common than these figures indicate.

Other Conditions Manifesting Bone Striations: Focal Dermal Hypoplasia

GOLTZ et al. (1962) delineated the syndrome of focal dermal hypoplasia in which areas of skin atrophy are associated with herniation of subcutaneous fat and linear pigmentation. Papillomata are found on the lips and anal margins, the nails are dysplastic, and the teeth are irregular. Syndactyly, clavicular defects and scoliosis are inconsistent features, and ocular abnormalities, microcephaly and mental retardation are sometimes encountered. The metaphyses of the long bones show well-marked longitudinal striations which are present in early infancy. The cranium is not sclerotic but variable structural defects may be evident in the extremities and other sites. The fact that bony striations are a component of the syndrome was established by LARRÉGUE et al. (1972) when they recognised these radiographic changes in 9 of a series of 11 children with focal dermal hypoplasia. The association of bone striations with focal dermal hypoplasia has been discussed by GORDON (1975) and CARLSON (1977).

In a review of 41 patients from the literature, GOLTZ et al. (1970) drew attention to the overwhelming female preponderance and gave a lengthy list of the many and varied skeletal anomalies which may occur in the syndrome. Focal dermal hypoplasia is probably inherited as an X-linked dominant, which is usually lethal in the male.

References

BLOOR DU (1954) A case of osteopathia striata. J Bone Joint Surg [Br] 36:261

DE BOER SM, VAN GOOL AV (1974) Schedet en gebitsafwijkingen bij een patiente met osteopathia striata. Ned Tijdschr Geneesk 118:1373

FAIRBANK HAT (1925) A case of unilateral affection of the skeleton of unknown origin. Br J Surg 12:594

FAIRBANK HAT (1950) Osteopathia striata. J Bone Joint Surg [Br] 32:117

FRANKLYN PP, WILKINSON D (1978) Two cases of osteopathia striata, deafness and cranial osteopetrosis. Ann Radiol (Paris) 21:91

GORDON W (1975) Focal dermal hypoplasia syndrome. S Afr Med J 15:287

HORAN FT, BEIGHTON PH (1978) Osteopathia striata with cranial sclerosis. An autosomal dominant entity. Clin Genet 13:201

HURT RL (1953) Osteopathia striata – Voorhoeve's disease. J Bone Joint Surg [Br] 35:89

JONES MD, MULCAHY ND (1968) Osteopathia striata, osteopetrosis and impaired hearing. Arch Otolaryngol 87:116

LARRÉGUE M, MAROTEAUX P, MICHEL Y, FAURÉ C (1972) L'ostéopathie striée, symptôme radiologique de l'hypoplasie dermique en aires. Ann Radiol (Paris) 15:287

RUCKER TN, ALFIDI T (1964) A rare familial affectation of the skeleton: Fairbank's disease. Radiology 82:63

TAYBI H, NUROCK AB (1969) Discussion of osteopathia striata. Birth Defects 5/4:105

VOORHOEVE N (1924) L'image radiologique non encore décrite d'une anomalie du squelette. Acta Radiol (Stockh) 3:407

WALKER B (1969) Osteopathia striata with cataracts and deafness. Birth Defects 5/4:295

Focal dermal hypoplasia

CARLSON DH (1977) Osteopathia striata revisited. J Can Assoc Radiol 28/3:190

GOLTZ RW, PETERSEN NC, GORLIN RJ, RAVITS HG (1962) Focal dermal hypoplasia. Arch Dermatol 86:708

GOLTZ RW, HENDERSON RR, HICH JM, OH JE (1970) Focal dermal hypoplasia syndrome. Arch Dermatol 101:1

GORDON W (1975) Focal dermal hypoplasia syndrome. S Afr Med J 49:1097

LARRÉGUE M, MAROTEAUX P, MICHEL Y, FAURE C (1972) L'ostéopathie striée, symptôme radiologique de l'hypoplasie dermique en aires. Ann Radiol (Paris) 15:287

Longitudinal sclerotic streaks in long bones may be found in isolation or in association with conditions of bony condensation such as osteopoikilosis or melorheostosis. There are, however, two syndromes in which bone striations are a significant component

I. Osteopathia striata with cranial sclerosis
Female aged 18 years (Horan and Beighton 1978)

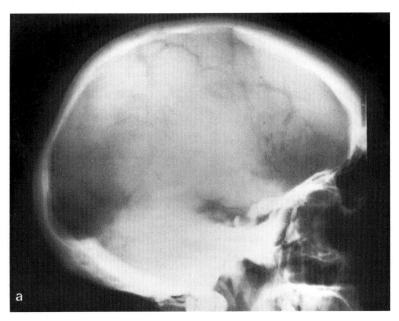

Case I

Fig. 15-1. (a) Skull. Sclerosis is evident in the base

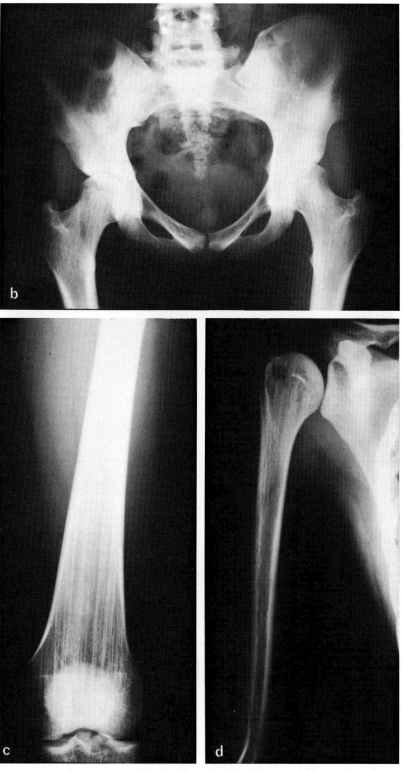

Fig. 15-1. (b) Pelvis. Fan-like sclerotic streaks are present in the iliac bones and femoral necks. (c and d) Femur and humerus. Longitudinal linear striations traverse the growth plates and shafts of the tubular bones

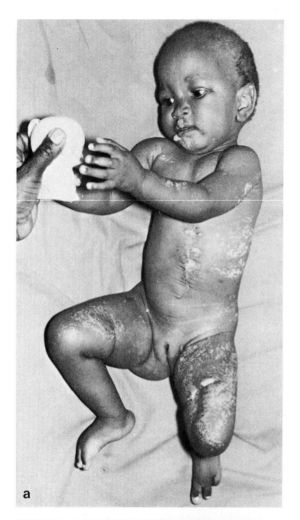

II. Focal Dermal Hypoplasia (Goltz Syndrome)
In addition to bone striations, the radiological
manifestations of this condition are numerous and
include hypoplasia of the vertebrae, clavicles, ribs
and pelvis, and malformations of the extremities.
This case is presented by courtesy of
Dr W. Gordon of Groote Schuur Hospital, Cape
Town

Case II
Infant aged 1 year (Gordon 1975)

Fig. 15-2. (a) The characteristic dermal
hypopigmentation, atrophy, and papillomata are
present, and the left foot is malformed

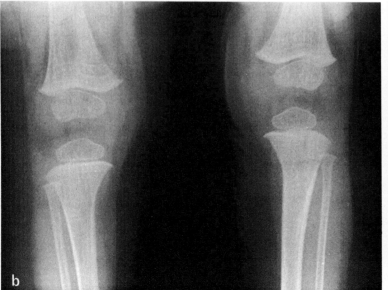

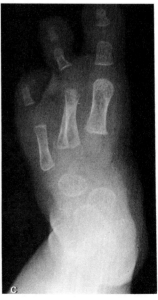

Fig. 15-2. (b) Knees. Linear striations are evident in the metaphyses

Fig. 15-2. (c) Foot. Many
bones are absent

Chapter 16

Osteopoikilosis

Historical and Nosological Considerations

Osteopoikilosis or 'spotted bones' is a benign condition in which multiple sclerotic foci are associated with patches of lentil-like papules in the skin. STIEDA (1905) is credited with the first description of osteopoikilosis, and LEDOUX-LEBARD et al. (1916) subsequently coined the term *osteopoecilie* from the Greek word *poikilos*, meaning spotted or mottled. VOORHOEVE (1924) recognised the familial nature of the condition, and WINDHOLZ (1932) noted the associated skin lesions, which he termed 'dermatofibrosis lenticularis disseminata.' HARMSTON (1956) also drew attention to these inconsistent dermal changes, employing the alternative designation 'osteopathia condensans disseminata' for the bone changes. In other reports, the terms 'osteitis condensans' and 'osteosclerosis generalisata disseminata' have been employed.

MELNICK (1959) reported two parents with the condition who produced eight children, all of whom were affected. GREEN et al. (1962) emphasised the difference between osteopoikilosis and melorheostosis (see Chap. 17) and RAQUE and WOOD (1970) discussed the dermatological features. In a comprehensive review, SZABO (1971) was able to find 300 cases in the literature.

Clinical Features

Osteopoikilosis usually remains clinically silent, and the diagnosis is most often made by chance when the bony manifestations are recognised after radiographic investigation for some unrelated purpose.

The dermal changes are present in about 10% of affected individuals and consist of patches of small, firm, yellowish papules. These lesions, 'dermatofibrosis lenticularis disseminata' are variable in quantity and distribution and may be entirely absent.

Both the bone and the skin lesions are usually static, although progression and disappearance have been reported. Concurrent osteosarcoma of the tibia has been reported in an affected 48-year-old male (MINDELL et al. 1978). This is the only instance of apparent malignant transformation and the risk of this hazard seems to be very low.

Radiographic Manifestations

The condition mainly affects the appendicular skeleton. Multiple, small, sharply demarcated sclerotic foci are distributed symmetrically in the metaphyses and epiphyses of the tubular bones and in the carpus and tarsus. The diaphyses are spared. The pelvis may be involved, but the skull, mandible, spine and thoracic cage are not affected.

The opacities vary in size but are 5 to 50 mm in diameter and may be very numerous. Whether they are age-related has not been clearly established, and they may enlarge, regress, or remain static for many years.

Comment

Osteopoikilosis is a harmless entity and its main importance lies in the differential diagnosis from other, more serious conditions. The multiplicity of the bony lesions in osteopoikilosis distinguishes them from solitary bone islands, and their well-defined outlines and distribution in symmetrically localised areas rule out osteoblastic metastases, tuberous sclerosis, and bone infarcts.

Areas of patchy sclerosis, especially in the epiphyses and bones of the carpus and tarsus, are seen in melorheostosis and may mimic osteopoikilosis. However, the additional longitudinal 'candle wax' sclerosis in the diaphyses, the lack of symmetry, the sclerodermatous skin changes, and the non-genetic aetiology of melorheostosis readily permit differentiation between the two entities.

References

GREEN AE, ELLSWOOD WH, COLLINS JR (1962) Melorheostosis and osteopoikilosis: with review of literature. A J R 87:1096

HARMSTON GJ (1956) Osteopathia condensans disseminata. Radiology 66:556

LEDOUX-LEBARD R, CHABANIX, DESSANE (1916) L'osteopoecilie, form nouvelle d'osteite condensante generalisée. J Radiol Electrol 2:133

MINDELL ER, NORTHUP CS, DOUGLASS HO (1978) Osteosarcoma associated with osteopoikilosis: Case report. J Bone Joint Surg [Am] 60:406

MELNICK JC (1959) Osteopathia condensans disseminata (osteopoikilosis). Study of a family of 4 generations. A J R 82:229

RAQUE CJ, WOOD MG (1970) Connective tissue naevus. Dermatofibrosis lenticularis disseminata with osteopoikilosis. Arch Dermatol 102:390

STIEDA A (1905) Über umschriebene Knochenvernichtungen in Bereich der Substantia spongiosa im Roentgenbilde. Beitr Klin Chir 45:700

SZABO AD (1971) Osteopoikilosis in a twin. Clin Orthop 79:156

VOORHOEVE N (1924) L'image radiologique non encore décrite d'une anomalie du squelette. Acta Radiol (Stockh) 3:407

WINDHOLZ F (1932) Über familäre Osteopoikilie und Dermatofibrosis lenticularis disseminata. Fortschr Roentgenstr 45:566

Osteopoikilosis is often diagnosed by chance. The features are well known and confusion with other conditions rarely arises

Case I
Male aged 30 years

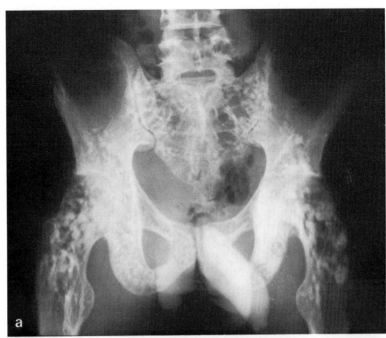

Fig. 16-1. (a) Pelvis. Multiple sclerotic lesions overlie each other and give the appearance of being confluent

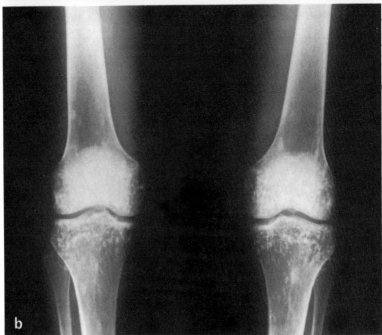

Fig. 16-1. (b) Knees. Typical changes in the ends of the femora and tibiae

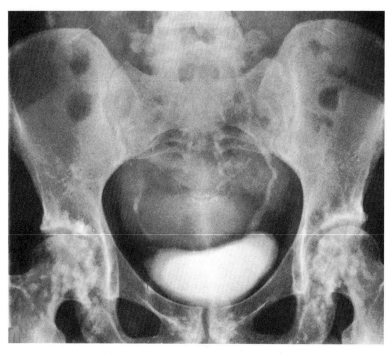

Case II
Male aged 68 years

Fig. 16-2. Pelvis. Numerous dense foci were observed incidently in the hip region during excretory urography. Their well-defined and regular appearance distinguishes them from neoplastic metastases

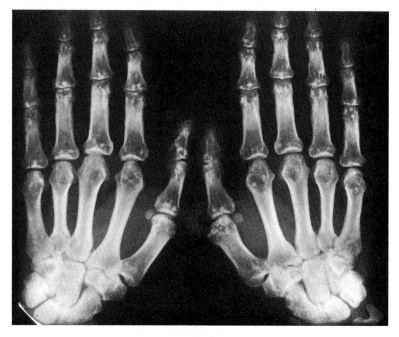

Case III
Female aged 34 years

Fig. 16-3. Hands. Multiple well-demarcated sclerotic lesions are seen in the carpus and at the ends of the tubular bones

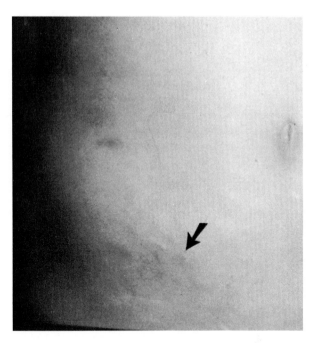

Case IV

Boy aged 14 years (the son of the patient shown in Fig. 16-3

Fig. 16-4. An indurated area of dermatofibrosis lenticularis disseminata is present in the right lower quadrant of the abdomen (arrow). This dermal abnormality is an inconstant concomitant of osteopoikilosis

Chapter 17

Melorheostosis

Historical and Nosological Considerations

LÉRI and JOANNI (1922) described a 39-year-old woman who had 'hyperostosis flowing along the whole length of the limb.' Subsequently LÉRI and LIÈVRE (1928) termed the condition 'melorheostosis' from the Greek *melos*, a limb, and *rheos*, a stream.

Numerous reports followed and it became apparent that the disorder had important clinical consequences. GREEN et al. (1962) discussed the distinction between melorheostosis and osteopoikilosis, and CAMPBELL et al. (1968) reviewed the clinical, radiographic and pathological findings in 14 cases.

WAGERS et al. (1972) considered the condition from the dermatological standpoint and SOFFA et al. (1975) mentioned that about 5% of patients have linear skin lesions overlying the affected bone. In a review of the literature, BEAUVAIS et al. (1977) commented that about 200 cases had been described. MURRAY (1978) discussed the features of 30 patients, whose ages ranged from 2 to 76 years, and pointed out that the distribution of the skeletal changes often corresponds to the anatomical arrangement of the sclerotomes. On this basis, he suggested that melorheostosis might be the end result of a sensory nerve lesion.

Clinical Features

Melorheostosis is a slowly progressive disorder which usually presents in late childhood. The manifestations are variable, and the diagnosis may be made by chance following radiographic investigation of obscure skeletal discomfort, limb deformities, or dermal lesions.

In contrast to the majority of sclerosing bone dysplasias, melorheostosis may cause considerable bone pain. This symptom is most common in adulthood and is precipitated by activity or fatigue. Disturbed bone growth in childhood can lead to limb-length discrepancy and secondary problems, including genu valgum and scoliosis.

The skin over the affected bones may be sclerodermatous or indurated and erythematous. The subcutaneous tissues and muscles may be involved and soft-tissue contractures may compound the patient's disability. In some individuals with melorheostosis these changes are severe; in others they are entirely absent.

The simultaneous occurrence of arteriovenous aneurysms and melorheostosis was observed by MURRAY (1951) and PATRICK (1969). Isolated reports of concomitant neurofibromatous and tuberous sclerosis are of doubtful significance and there are no other systemic ramifications. Neither pathological fractures nor malignant degeneration have been reported.

Radiographic Manifestations

The classical radiographic feature of melorheostosis in adulthood is heaped-up sclerotic bone which gives the appearance of wax flowing down the side of a candle. In childhood the hyperostosis does not extend beyond the boundaries of the cortex, and external contours of the bone are not disturbed.

Skull, Spine, Chest, and Pelvis

Involvement of the skull, spine and thoracic cage is rare, but when the flat bones are affected, the sclerosis is irregular and patchy. In the pelvis sclerosis is maximal around the acetabula and it may extend across the ilia in a streaky, fan-shaped configuration.

Limbs

The tubular bones are the site of predilection and the lower limbs are more frequently involved than the arms. The abnormalities are usually limited to a single bone or limb and sometimes skip a segment. They may be bilateral, but involvement is never symmetrical.

The longitudinal density encroaches upon the medullary cavity, and usually only one side of the bone is affected. In adults the linear density extends beyond the cortex in multiple periosteal outgrowths, which give the 'flowing wax' appearance. Involvement of an epiphysis may be partial but sclerosis may be complete in the small bones of the carpus and tarsus. There may be premature closure of the epiphyseal plate, with unequal growth of an affected limb. Ectopic bone may form in adjacent soft tissues, and bony outgrowths within the joints may limit movement.

Comment

The aetiology of melorheostosis is unknown. Males and females are affected with equal frequency; there is no familial tendency and no evidence to indicate a genetic basis.

Sophisticated techniques which have been employed in an attempt to determine the basic defect include bone scanning with technetium-labelled polyphosphate (BIED et al. 1976), measurement of bone density by photon absorption, and assessment of blood circulation by the ^{133}Xenon clearance method (PAJARINEN et al. 1978). These latter authors reached the conclusion that there is no systemic disturbance in calcium metabolism, although blood flow is increased and metabolic activity is accelerated in the regions involved.

In spite of these investigations, it is still debatable whether melorheostosis is the consequence of primary vascular or neurological factors or whether it represents a connective-tissue abiotrophy or a localised defect in embryogenesis.

References

BEAUVAIS P, FAURÉ C, MONTAGNE J-P, CHIGOT PL, MAROTEAUX P (1977) Leri's melorheostosis: Three pediatric cases and a review of the literature. Pediatr Radiol 6:153

BIED JC, MALSH C, MEUNIER P (1976) La mélorhéostose chez l'adulte. Rev Rhum Mal Ostéoartic 43:193

CAMPBELL CJ, PAPADEMETRIOU T, BONFIGLIO M (1968) Melorheostosis: A report of the clinical, roentgenographic and pathological findings in fourteen cases. J Bone Joint Surg 50:1281

GREEN AE, ELWOOD WH, COLLINS JR (1962) Melorheostosis and osteopoikilosis, with a review of the literature. A J R 87:1096

LÉRI A, JOANNI J (1922) Une affection non décrite des os: hyperostose 'en coulée' sur toute la longueur d'un membre ou mélorhéostose. Bull Soc Méd Hôp Paris 46:1141

LÉRI A, LIÈVRE JA (1928) La mélorhéostose (hyperostose d'un membre en coulée). Presse Méd 36:801

MURRAY RO (1951) Melorheostosis associated with congenital arteriovenous aneurysms. Proc R Soc Med 44:473

MURRAY RO (1978) Sclerotome theory of melorheostosis. Proceedings of the 5th Annual Meeting of the International Skeletal Society. Boston. Case 26, p 9

PAJARINEN P, ALHAVA E, REHNBERG V (1978) Melorheostosis. A case report with special reference to bone mineral density, bone circulation and bone scan. Ann Chir Gynaecol 67:36

PATRICK JH (1969) Melorheostosis associated with arterio-venous aneurysm of the left arm and trunk: A report of a case with a long follow-up. J Bone Joint Surg [Br] 51:126

SOFFA DJ, SIRE DJ, DODSON JH (1975) Melorheostosis with linear sclerodermatous skin changes. Radiology 114:577

WAGERS LT, YOUNG AW, RYAN SF (1972) Linear melorheostotic scleroderma. Br J Dermatol 86:297

.

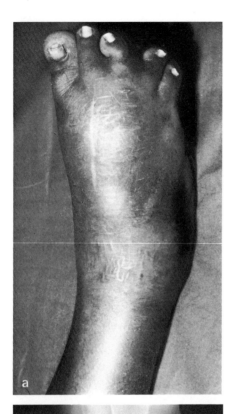

Case I
Female aged 48 years

Fig. 17-1. (a) The soft tissues
overlying the bone lesions are tense
and indurated. (b and c) Leg.
There are irregular linear densities
along the fibula and the tarsal
bones

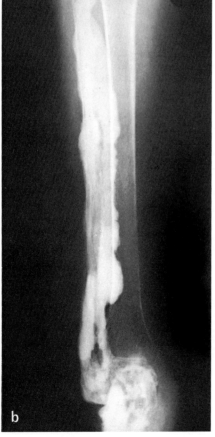

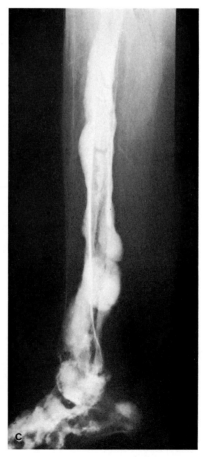

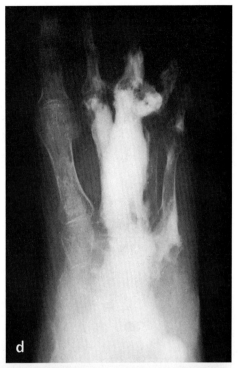

Fig. 17-1. (d and e) Foot. The characteristic 'flowing molten wax' appearance is evident

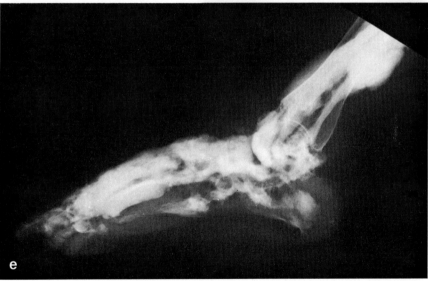

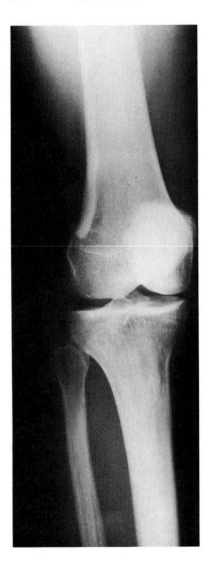

Case II
Female, aged 16 years

Fig. 17-2. Knee. The changes in this patient are much less florid and the sclerotic linear lesion is seen only on the lateral aspect of the lower femur

Chapter 18

Osteoectasia
with Hyperphosphatasia

Historical and Nosological Considerations

Although fewer than 30 cases have been reported, this condition has enjoyed numerous designations. The first report emanated from BAKWIN and EIGER (1956), following their study of a Puerto Rican girl with 'fragile bones and macrocranium.' BAKWIN et al. (1964) subsequently described her affected sisters under the title 'osteoectasia with macrocranium,' and other sets of siblings with the condition from the same Caribbean island were reported by EYRING and EISENBERG (1968) and by THOMPSON et al. (1969) as having 'congenital or hereditary hyperphosphatasia.'

The resemblance of the radiographic changes to those of the common adult form of Paget disease was noted by CHOREMIS et al. (1958) and SWOBODA (1958), and the terms 'osteitis deformans' and 'hyperostosis corticalis deformans juvenalis' were used in the titles of their papers. In a study of an affected boy in England, MARSHALL (1962) observed that the serum alkaline phosphatase level was elevated and drew attention to this fact by entitling his article 'chronic progressive osteopathy with hyperphosphatasia.'

The term 'osteoectasia with hyperphosphatasia' is employed in the Paris Nomenclature and in recent reports some form of the designation 'hyperphosphatasia' has been preferred. For the sake of clarity, this latter term is used throughout this chapter.

Although hyperphosphatasia is rare, patients have been reported from many parts of the world and in diverse ethnic groups. Published cases, their authors, designations, and the geographical derivations of subjects are shown in Table 18-1.

Clinical Features

The condition has its onset in the first three years of life and affected children experience episodes of pyrexia and bone pain. The skull enlarges, the long bones become bowed, and pathological fractures add to the stunting of stature and deformity. Optic atrophy and deafness are late complications. Angioid streaks may be present in the retina. These ribbon-like lesions, which underlie the blood vessels, are the result of breaks in Bruch's

Table 18-1. Osteoectasia with hyperphosphatasia – published cases

Author	Designation	Patient	Geographical derivation
BAKWIN and EIGER (1956)	Fragile bones with macrocranium	Girl, 7[a]	Puerto Rico
CHOREMIS et al. (1958)	Osteitis deformans (Paget's disease)	Boy, 12	Greece
SWOBODA (1958)	Hyperostosis corticalis deformans juvenilis	2 Infant sisters[a]	Austria
MARSHALL (1962)	Chronic progressive osteopathy with hyperphosphatasia	Boy and infant	England
BAKWIN et al. (1964)	Familial osteoectasia with macrocranium	Sisters of patient of BAKWIN and EIGER (1956)[a]	Puerto Rico
FANCONI et al. (1964)	Osteochalasia desmalis familiaris	Boy and infant	Brazil
EYRING and EISENBERG (1968)	Congenital hyperphosphatasia	Brother and sister infants	Puerto Rico
THOMPSON et al. (1969)	Hereditary hyperphosphatasia	Sister and 2 brothers	Puerto Rico
WOODHOUSE et al. (1972)	Paget's disease	Child, 5	United Kingdom
CAFFEY (1973)	Familial hyperphosphatasemia with ateliosis	i) Infant girl ii) 7 Children in 2 families	U.S.A. Puerto Rico
DESAI et al. (1973)	Chronic idiopathic hyperphosphatasia	Infant boy[a]	India
FRETZIN (1975)	Hyperphosphatasia	Girl, 12	U.S.A.
WHALEN et al. (1977)	Bone dysplasia with hyperphosphatasia	Brother, 4 sister, 7	Guatemala
DUILLO et al. (1977)	Chronic idiopathic hyperphosphatasia	Girl, 2	Italy

[a] Consanguinity.

membrane and are also found in Paget disease and pseudoxanthoma elasticum. As in other skeletal dysplasias in which metabolic activity in bone is increased, the serum alkaline phosphatase levels are raised. Hyperphosphatasia is a progressive disease and fatal complications due to arterial involvement have been described. As there are no reports of adults with the disorder, it is reasonable to assume that the prognosis is uniformly bad. However, calcitonin therapy might prove to be of value (WOODHOUSE et al. 1972; WHALEN et al. 1977).

Radiographic Manifestations

Radiographic changes are most marked in the skull and limbs. There is some similarity in appearance to the combined active and reparative stages of the adult form of Paget disease. The pattern is that of lack of architecturally normal cortical bone due to abnormal bone resorption (BLANC 1978). The radiographic features have been reviewed by CAFFEY (1973).

Skull

The calvarium is thickened, and irregular dense areas which have been likened to 'cotton-wool balls' are seen in the vault. The facial bones are not affected to any extent.

Spine, Pelvis, and Chest

Softening of the bones may lead to platyspondyly and protrusio acetabuli. The flat bones show diffuse widening with 'cystic' changes and sclerosis.

Limbs

The tubular bones are increased in girth due to layers of poorly formed cortical bone in their shafts. The bone has a coarse trabecular pattern and the medullary cavities are widened. The overall appearance may be that of osteoporosis, with streaky areas of density. The weight-bearing bones often become bowed.

Comment

The yellow 'cobblestone' dermal changes of pseudoxanthoma elasticum (PXE) have been reported in at least two children with hyperphosphatasia (MITSUDO 1971; FRETZIN 1975). Retinal angioid streaks which occur in hyperphosphatasia are also a feature of PXE and the adult form of Paget disease. For these reasons, it is possible that the three conditions might share a common pathogenic mechanism.

There are several examples of affected sibs (EYRING and EISENBERG 1968; THOMPSON et al. 1969; WHALEN et al. 1977) or parental consanguinity (BAKWIN and EIGER 1956; SWOBODA 1958; DESAI et al. 1973) and inheritance is evidently autosomal recessive. However, there is considerable variation in severity and hyperphosphatasia may be heterogeneous. A report of an affected mother and daughter is certainly suggestive of dominant inheritance and genetic heterogeneity (FRETZIN 1975).

References

BAKWIN H, EIGER MS (1956) Fragile bones and macrocranium. J Pediatr 49:558
BAKWIN H, GOLDEN A, FOX S (1964) Familial osteoectasia with macrocranium. A J R 91:609

CAFFEY J (1973) Familial hyperphosphatasemia with ateliosis and hypermetabolism of growing membranous bone. Review of the clinical, radiographic and chemical features. In: KAUFMANN HJ (ed) Intrinsic diseases of bones. Karger, Basel (Progress in pediatric radiology, vol 4, p 438)

CHOREMIS C, YANNAKOS D, PAPADATOS C, BAROUTSOU E (1958) Osteitis deformans (Paget's disease) in an 11 year-old boy. Helv Paediatr Acta 13:185

DESAI MP, JOSHI NC, SHAH KN (1973) Chronic idiopathic hyperphosphatasia in an Indian child. Am J Dis Child 126:626

DUILLO MT, PELIZZA A, CARAMIA G (1977) Chronic idiopathic hyperphosphatasia. Panminerva Med 19:53

EYRING EJ, EISENBERG E (1968) Congenital hyperphosphatasia. J Bone Joint Surg [Am] 50:1099

FANCONI G, MOREIRA G, UEHLINGER E, GIEDION A (1964) Osteochalasia desmalis familiaris. Helv Paediatr Acta 19:279

FRETZIN DF (1975) Pseudoxanthoma elasticum in hyperphosphatasia. Arch Dermatol 111:271

MARSHALL WC (for MONCRIEFF AA) (1962) Chronic progressive osteopathy with hyperphosphatasia. Proc R Soc Med 55:238

MITSUDO SM (1971) Chronic idiopathic hyperphosphatasia associated with pseudoxanthoma elasticum. J Bone Joint Surg [Am] 53:303

SWOBODA W (1958) Hyperostosis corticalis deformans juvenilis. Helv Paediatr Acta 13:292

THOMPSON RC JR, GAUL GE, HORWITZ SJ, SCHENK RK (1969) Hereditary hyperphosphatasia. Study of 3 siblings. Am J Med 47:209

WHALEN JP, HORWITH M, KROOK L, MACINTYRE I, MENA E, VITERI F, TORUN B, NUNEZ EA (1977) Calcitonin treatment in hereditary bone dysplasia with hyperphosphatasemia: A radiographic and histologic study of bone. A J R 129:29

WOODHOUSE NJY, FISHER MT, SIGURDSSON G, JOPLIN GF, MACINTYRE I (1972) Paget's disease in a 5-year-old: Acute response to human calcitonin. Br Med J 4:267

This case, presented by courtesy of Dr W.E. Berdon of the Presbyterian Hospital, New York, illustrates the condition in a 19-year-old Puerto Rican girl (Thompson et al. 1969)

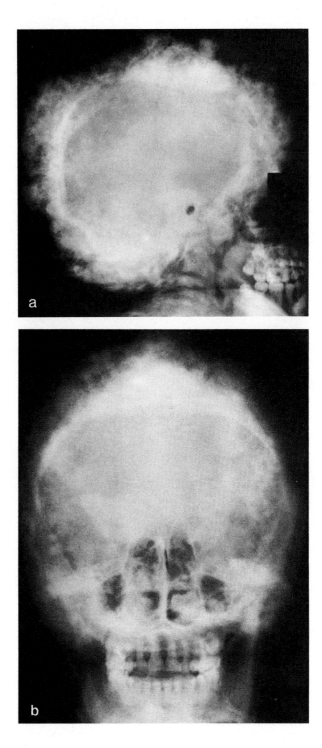

Fig. 18-1 a and b. Frontal and lateral views of the skull. There is enormous uneven thickening of the calvarium, which contains numerous round patches that resemble cotton-wool balls. By contrast, the facial bones appear normal

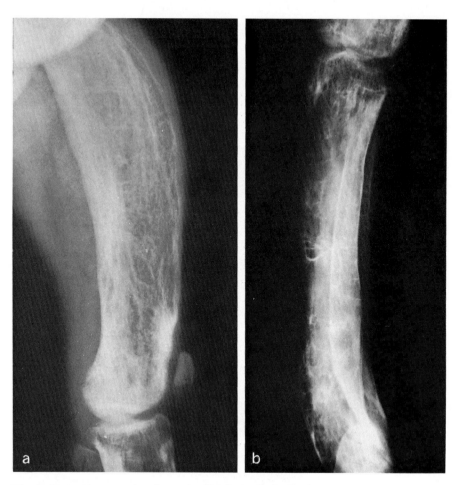

Fig. 18-2 a and b. Lateral radiograph of left lower limb. The bones are bowed and enlarged. The opaque transverse lines are suggestive of microfractures

Chapter 19

Infantile Cortical Hyperostosis (Caffey Disease)

Historical and Nosological Considerations

Although early accounts of infantile cortical hyperostosis were associated with the names of RöSKE, DE TONI, SMYTH, CAFFEY, and SILVERMAN, the definitive description by CAFFEY (1946) gave the condition its eponym.

The disorder has a world-wide distribution and occurs in all strata of society. The usual acute form presents in the first five months of life and regresses completely. The rare 'juvenile' form may follow a longer course. It is considered by many to represent late recurrence in a previously unrecognised case, with reactivation of persistent lesions (BLANK 1975; FRÁNÂ and SEKANINA 1976).

Clinical Features

Caffey disease has many characteristics of an inflammatory disorder. The tubular bones, shoulder girdle and mandible are most frequently involved, and hard, tender, soft-tissue swellings are associated with pyrexia, leucocytosis and a raised erythrocyte sedimentation rate.

Swelling precedes the radiological changes, is not associated with erythema or heat, and may be accompanied by limitation of movement in the extremities. The mandible is involved in about 80% of patients, usually, but not invariably, in association with other bones (FAURÉ et al. 1977). FINSTERBUSH and RANG (1975) have documented the features and course in 29 cases.

Radiographic Manifestations

The main radiographic change is marked hyperostosis, and new bone formation produces irregular widening of the cortices of the affected bones. The clinical and radiographic features have been reviewed by CAFFEY (1957).

Skull

The mandible and zygoma are predominantly affected. The mandibular lesions are variable but usually florid and bilateral. In the early stages it may be difficult to recognise bone involvement under the soft-tissue swelling. After two or three weeks it is usually evident that the bones are thickened, with a uniform ground-glass appearance. The bony outline is initially ill-defined, but later a thin, sometimes stratified margin is discernible. These changes are often bilateral. In the skull vault there are no conspicuous features although small lytic lesions have been reported (BOYD, SHAW and THOMAS, 1972).

Spine

The spine is not affected.

Chest and Pelvis

Involvement of the clavicles and scapulae is common and frequently unilateral. In the ribs the cortical hyperostosis is seen most prominently in the lateral arcs. Peripheral hyperostosis of the ilial wings is limited inferiorly by the acetabula.

Limbs

The changes in the tubular bones are frequently asymmetrical, with unequal involvement and even non-involvement of bones in the same limb. The metaphyses or epiphyses are never affected and the small round bones of the extremities are spared. The subperiosteal cortical enlargement may initially be homogeneous, but as the condition progresses, lamination becomes evident and pronounced coarse marginal irregularities of the cortex may develop.
In the chronic and recurrent forms resorption of endosteal bone occurs. In this way, the bones become wide, but thin-walled, with enlarged medullary cavities. These bones are eventually remodelled but deformities may persist, including mandibular asymmetry and interosseous bridges between the long bones.

Comment

The aetiology of the condition is unknown, although fetal damage, infection, allergy and genetic transmission have all been incriminated. At one time CAFFEY (1975) favoured the concept of infection, as this would explain the pathological features of a subperiosteal inflammatory reaction in the acute phase (EVERSOLE et al. 1957). Sporadic outbreaks in different geographic areas have occurred (CAFFEY 1975; CREMIN 1979).

Cases are usually sporadic, but there have been several instances of familial clustering (TAMPAS et al. 1960; PAJEWSKI and VURE 1957). FRÁNÂ and SEKANINA (1976) collected data concerning 11 patients in two generations of a kindred and postulated that genetic transmission might be autosomal dominant with varying expressivity. There have been two reports of diagnosis in utero in late pregnancy (BARBA and FRERIKS 1953; BENNETT and NELSON 1953).

The radiographic recognition of the acute variety of CAFFEY disease usually presents little difficulty. Vitamin A intoxication and scurvy produce a subperiosteal reaction in the long bones but are unlikely to occur before the age of six months. The jaw involvement and lack of metaphyseal lesions distinguish it from syphilis and the battered child syndrome.

References

BARBA WP, FRERIKS DJ (1953) The familial occurrence of infantile cortical hyperostosis in utero. J Pediatr 42:141

BENNETT HS, NELSON TR (1953) Prenatal cortical hyperostosis. Br J Radiol 26:47

BLANK E (1975) Recurrent Caffey's cortical hyperostosis and persistent deformity. Pediatrics 55:856

BOYD RDM, SHAW DG, THOMAS BM (1972) Infantile cortical hyperostosis with lytic lesions in the skull. Arch Dis Child 47:471

CAFFEY J (1946) Infantile cortical hyperostoses. J Pediat 29:541

CAFFEY J (1957) Infantile cortical hyperostosis; A review of the clinical and radiographic features. Proc R Soc Med 50:347

CREMIN BJ (1979) Caffey's disease in Cape Town. S Afr Med J 55:377

EVERSOLE SL, HOLMAN GH, ROBINSON RA (1957) Hitherto undescribed characteristics of the pathology of infantile cortical hyperostosis (Caffey's disease). Bull Johns Hopkins Hosp 101:80

FAURÉ C, BEYSSAC JM, MONTAGNE JP (1977) Predominant or exclusive orbital and facial involvement in infantile cortical hyperostosis (de Toni-Caffey's disease). Report of four cases and a review of the literature. Pediatr Radiol 6:103

FINSTERBUSH A, RANG M (1975) Infantile cortical hyperostosis. Follow up of 29 cases. Acta Orthop Scand 46:727

FRÁNÂ L, SEKANINA M (1976) Infantile cortical hyperostosis. Arch Dis Child 51:589

PAJEWSKI M, VURE E (1967) Late manifestations of infantile cortical hyperostosis. Br J Radiol 40:90

TAMPAS JP, VAN BUSKIRK FW, PETERSON OS (1960) Caffey's disease: Ten cases in two generations of one family. J A M A 172:1827

Many patients with infantile cortical hyperostosis probably go unrecognised, as the jaw enlargement is often insufficient to warrant radiological investigation. Although only one definite case had been reported in Southern Africa, six affected infants, including two Negro sisters, were seen at the Red Cross Children's Hospital, Cape Town during the period 1972–1976. The significant changes in three of these children are depicted (Case 1, 2 and 3) and the distribution of the lesions in all six is shown diagrammatically in Figure 19-4 (Cremin 1979)

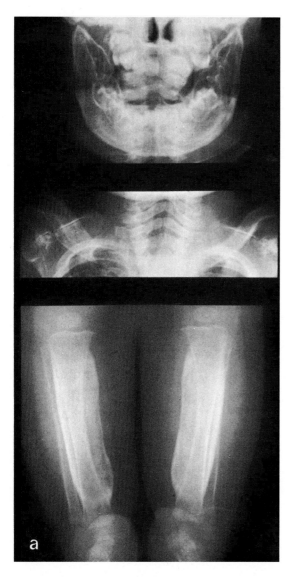

Case I
Female infant aged 5 months

Fig. 19-1. (a) Diffuse hyperostosis is seen in mandible, right clavicle and both tibiae. The hyperostotic cortex shows the typical ground-glass appearance. The mandible and clavicles, which are the first bones to develop, are predominantly involved

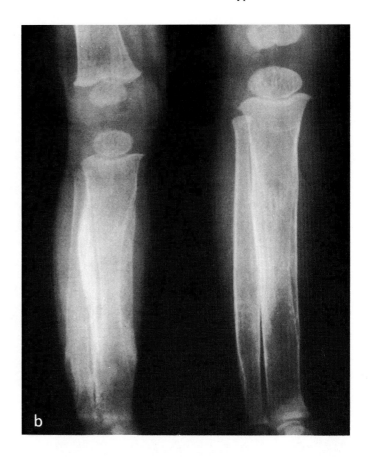

Fig. 19-1. (b) Aged 9 months.
The hyperostosis is resolving, but
changes persist in the right tibia, where
the cortex has an irregular outline

Case II
Sister of Case 1, aged 1 month

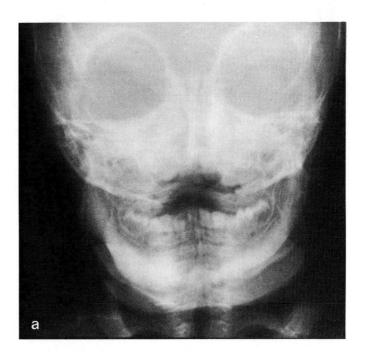

Fig. 19-2. (a) Hyperostotic changes are
present in the mandible

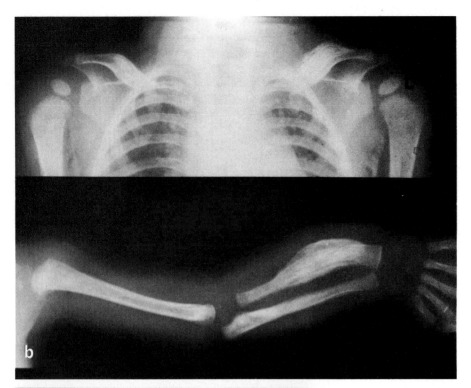

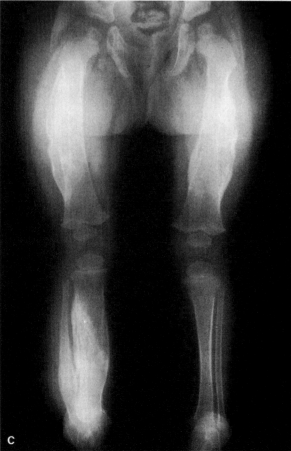

Fig. 19-2. (b) Clavicles and left arm. Changes are present in both clavicles and the radius is markedly involved. This patient demonstrates irregular involvement of bones in the same limb. A month later it became apparent that the ulna was also affected. (c) Lower limbs. The femora have homogeneous cortical hyperostosis and irregular outlines. The right tibia and fibula are affected; the left tibia and fibula are uninvolved

Case III
Infant aged 4 months

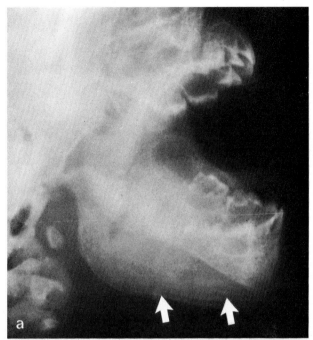

Fig. 19-3. (a) Subcortical lamination (arrows) may be a feature

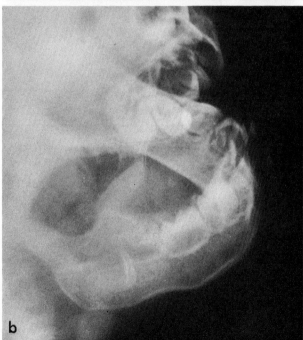

Fig. 19-3. (b) The mandible at 1 year of age. Resolution is complete, although the outline remains uneven

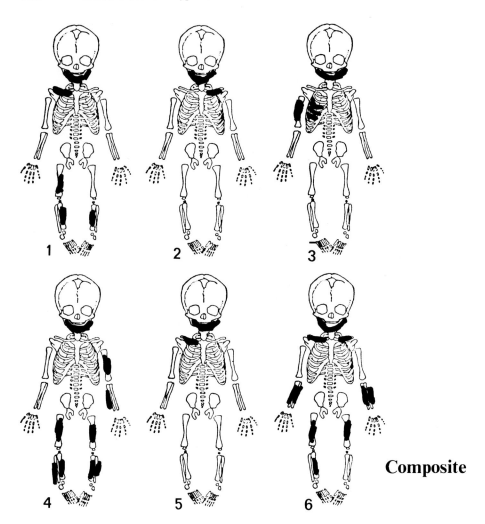

Composite

Fig. 19-4. The site of the lesions in six affected children. The authors have shown by a silver nitrate staining technique that the mandible and clavicle are amongst the first bones to show osseous development in the foetus. It is significant that these bones are the ones predominantly affected and indicates that the pathogenesis starts at an early age (8–10 weeks)

Chapter 20

Oculodento-Osseous Dysplasia

Historical and Nosological Considerations

GORLIN et al. (1963) delineated this condition, using the designation 'oculo-dentodigital dysplasia,' and pointed out that in addition to their patient, five others could be identified in the literature. Subsequently, REISNER et al. (1969) reviewed the features of 43 cases, and a decade later the number of reported patients had risen to more than 66 (SUGAR 1978).

There has been clinical and semantic confusion with similar disorders, including orodigitalfacial dysostosis, and this problem was compounded when O'ROURK and BRAVOS (1969) described an individual with the additional feature of pre-axial polydactyly, terming the condition 'oculodentodigital syndrome type II.' The nosological difficulties were partially resolved when the modified title 'oculodento-osseous dysplasia (ODOD)' was used in the 1970 Paris Nomenclature. This new appellation has found general favour but did not appear in the 1977 version of the Nomenclature.

Clinical Features

The major stigmata of ODOD are: microphthalmia; microcornea; a narrow nose with hypoplasia of the alae nasi and attenuated nostrils; fine, sparse hair; hypoplasia of the dental enamel; and, occasionally, cleft lip and palate. Secondary glaucoma may lead to blindness during childhood. Digital involvement is variable, but syndactyly of the fourth and fifth fingers is common; in those not affected in this way clinodactyly of the fifth finger is usually present.

Patients are of normal intelligence and physique, and apart from ocular disturbance many have enjoyed good health. However, there is a great variability in the severity of the skeletal manifestations and some affected individuals have been profoundly handicapped, with serious neurological impairment due to spinal cord compression at the base of the skull and facial distortion due to gross mandibular overgrowth.

Radiographic Manifestations

In many patients radiographic stigmata have been of minor degree, the changes consisting of mild undermodelling of the tubular bones and minor hyperostosis (LITTLEWOOD and LEWIS 1963; RAJIC and DE VEBER 1966). However, cranial sclerosis has been noted, and modelling defects may be marked (DAVID and PALMER 1958; COWAN 1959; PFEIFFER et al. 1968). These discrepancies may indicate heterogeneity, but so far this problem remains unresolved.

Skull

Apart from small orbits, involvement is variable; in some cases the calvarium and base are sclerotic. The mandible is broadened and may be massively enlarged, with an obtuse angle. The majority of patients are edentulous after adolescence.

Spine

The dorsal vertebrae may show some platyspondyly but the lumbar vertebrae are normal in shape.

Chest and Pelvis

There is widening of the medial portions of the clavicles and in extreme cases they present a 'pork chop' appearance. The ribs may also be slightly widened.
The pelvis is normal in configuration but may show mild sclerosis.

Limbs

Involvement of the tubular bones is mild, and is most evident in the distal portions of the radius and ulna. In some patients moderate cortical hyperostosis is present.
In the extremities syndactyly is common, particularly in the fourth and fifth fingers. Clinodactyly of the fifth finger due to a short middle phalanx is a consistent finding. In the feet the middle phalanges may be hypoplastic or absent.

Comment

ODOD is beset by semantic confusion, variable clinical expression, anomalous inheritance, and possible heterogeneity. The ocular, nasal and dental features are consistent but there are considerable discrepancies in the severity of cranial hyperostosis, mandibular overgrowth and digital involvement. Heterogeneity may exist at a genetic level: although the usual mild form of the disorder is inherited as an autosomal dominant, there is evidence to indicate that the severe variety depicted in this chapter might be inherited as an autosomal recessive (BEIGHTON et al. 1979).

In terms of differential diagnosis, the syndactyly and facial distortion may lead to confusion with sclerosteosis, while the medial clavicular expansion is reminiscent of Pyle disease. The characteristic changes in the eyes, nose and teeth serve to distinguish ODOD from these disorders.

References

BEIGHTON P, HAMERSMA H, RAAD M (1979) Oculodentoosseous dysplasia; heterogeneity or variable expression? Clin Genet 16:169

COWAN A (1959) Leontiasis ossea. Oral Surg 12:983

DAVID JEA, PALMER PES (1958) Familial metaphysial dysplasia. J Bone Joint Surg 40:86

GORLIN RJ, MESKIN LH, GEME JWST (1963) Oculodentodigital dysplasia. J. Pediatr 63:69

LITTLEWOOD JM, LEWIS GM (1963) The Holmes-Adie syndrome in a boy with acute juvenile rheumatism and bilateral syndactyly. Arch Dis Child 38:86

O'ROURK TR, BRAVOS A (1969) Oculo-dento-digital syndrome II. Birth Defects 5/2:226

PFEIFFER RA, ERPENSTEIN H, JUNEMANN G (1968) Oculo-dento-digitale Dysplasie. Klin. Monatsbl Augenheilk 152:247

RAJIC DS, DE VEBER LL (1966) Hereditary oculodentosseous dysplasia. Ann Radiol (Paris) 9:224

REISNER SH, KOTT E, BORNSTEIN B, SALINGER H, KAPLAN I, GORLIN RJ (1969) Oculodentodigital dysplasia. Am J Dis Child 118:600

SUGAR HS (1978) Oculodentodigital dysplasia syndrome with angle-closure glaucoma. Am J Ophthalmol 86:36

The patients depicted in this chapter are severely affected, unrelated males, aged 25 and 21, both of whom had blindness, facial distortion and quadriplegia. These two cases are atypical by virtue of the calcification of the basal ganglia, a complication which has many causes. The skull sclerosis, which is of unusual severity, may be age-related (Beighton et al. 1979). The skull radiographs and CT scans are published by courtesy of Professor J.C. de Villiers of Cape Town

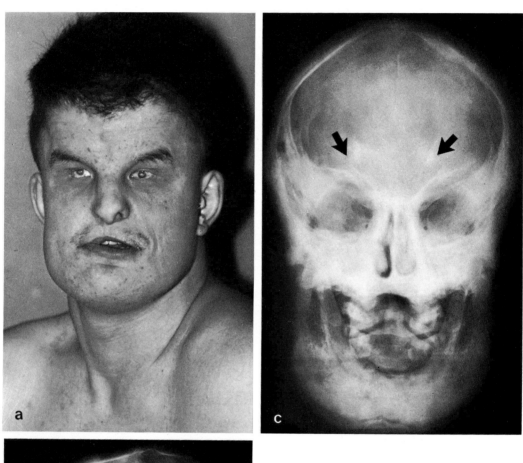

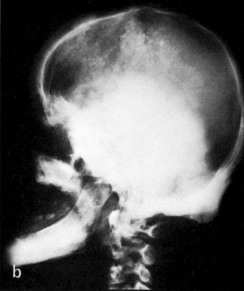

Case I
Male, aged 25 years

Fig. 20-1. (a) The eyes are small, the nose narrow, the hair sparse, and the mandible enlarged and asymmetrical. (b) Skull. Hyperostosis and sclerosis are present, especially in the occipitotemporal region, maxilla and mandible. (c) Skull. Massive asymmetric enlargement of the mandible is evident. Calcification is present in the basal ganglia (arrows)

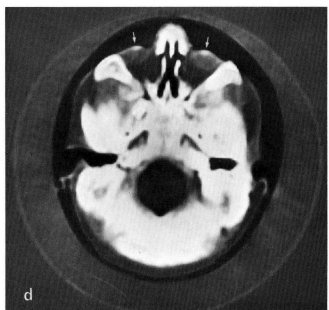

Fig. 20-1. (d) Skull. CT Scan. There is microphthalmia and calcification in the anterior region of the eye (arrows)

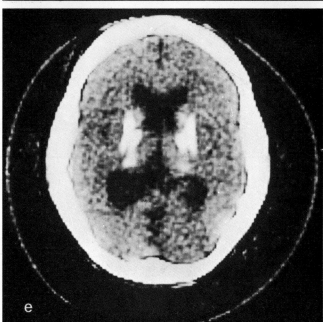

Fig. 20-1. (e) Skull. CT Scan. The ventricles are dilated and calcification of the basal ganglia is demonstrated

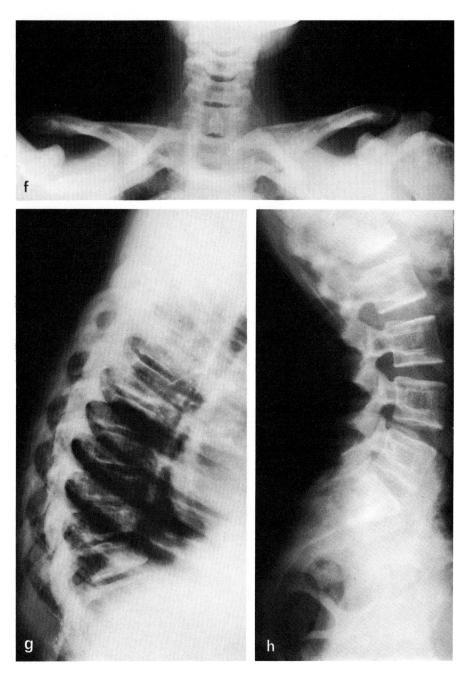

Fig. 20-1. (f) Clavicles. They are medially expanded with a 'pork chop' configuration.
(g) Spine (thoracic). The vertebral bodies show slight platyspondyly. (h) Spine (lumbar).
The configuration of the vertebral bodies is normal but there is central linear sclerosis

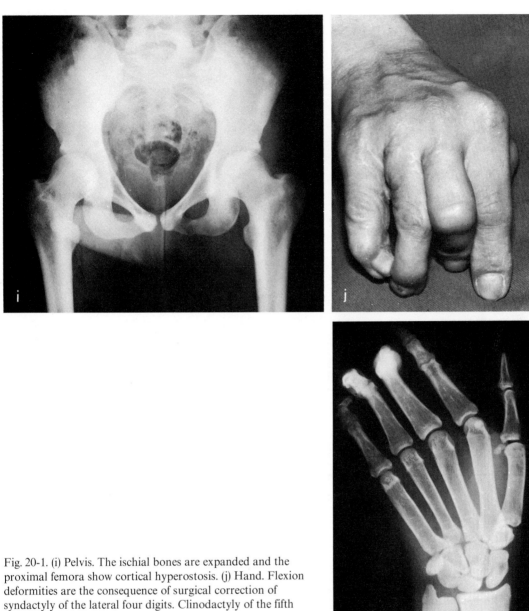

Fig. 20-1. (i) Pelvis. The ischial bones are expanded and the proximal femora show cortical hyperostosis. (j) Hand. Flexion deformities are the consequence of surgical correction of syndactyly of the lateral four digits. Clinodactyly of the fifth finger is a consistent feature of ODOD. (k) The middle phalynx of the fifth finger shows the typical cuboid configuration

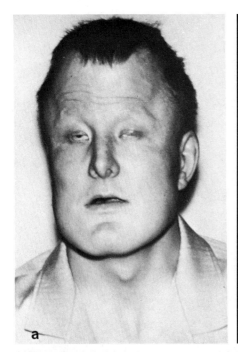

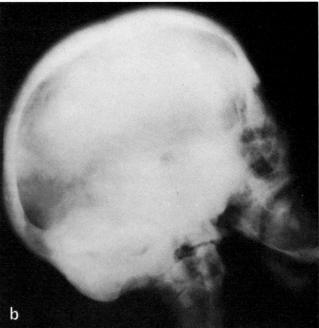

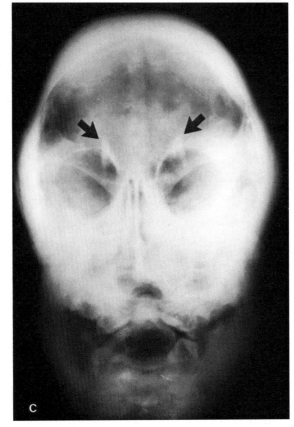

Case II
Male, aged 21 years

Fig. 20-2. (a) The facial appearance is very similar to that of the previous patient. Microphthalmia, nasal narrowing, sparsity of hair, and gross asymmetric mandibular enlargement are evident. (b) Skull. Calvarial hyperostosis and mandibular overgrowth are major features. (c) Skull. Generalised calvarial and maxillary sclerosis and calcification of the basal ganglia are evident (arrows)

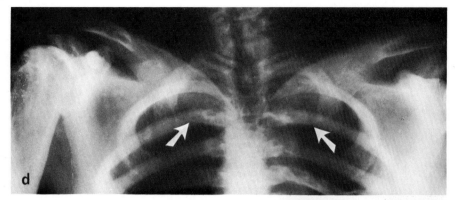

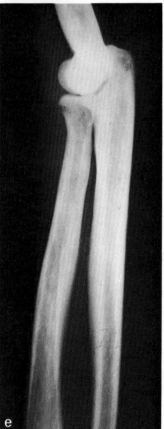

Fig. 20-2. (d) Chest. Expansion of the medial ends of the clavicles is extreme (arrows on lower borders). (e) Forearm. The cortices of the proximal radius and ulna are thickened

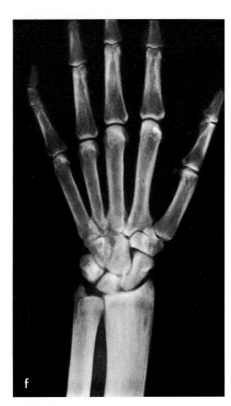

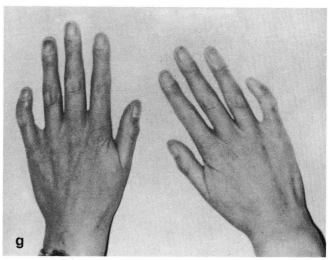

Fig. 20-2. (f) The fifth finger shows the characteristic hypoplasia of the middle phalynx. (g) Hand. The fifth fingers are short and incurved

Chapter 21

Miscellaneous Sclerosing Dysplasias

Bone sclerosis and hyperostosis are features of a number of conditions that warrant brief mention. The following are considered in this chapter:

1. Osteitis deformans (Paget disease)
2. Pachydermoperiostosis
3. Stanescu syndrome
4. Tubular stenosis (Kenny-Caffey syndrome)
5. Familial osteodysplasia
6. Schwarz-Lélek syndrome
7. Sclerotic bone-dentine dysplasia syndrome
8. Osteopetrosis with familial paraplegia
9. Central osteosclerosis with bamboo hair
10. Weismann-Netter-Stuhl syndrome (toxopachyostéose diaphysaire tibio-péronière)

1. Osteitis Deformans

Osteitis deformans, which was described by Sir James Paget in 1877, is the most common of the sclerosing bone dysplasias. The condition has a predilection for the Caucasian races and there are striking regional differences in prevalence. In the endemic areas, it is said to be present in more than 10% of persons over the age of 40 years (Nager 1975). Paget disease has been the subject of extensive reviews (Brailsford 1954; Barry 1969; Guyer and Clough 1978), and the manifestations are so well known that detailed description in this chapter is not warranted.

Although about 20% of patients with osteitis deformans are asymptomatic and only diagnosed incidentally, the usual clinical presentation is progressive bone pain, nerve compression from distortion in the skull and vertebrae, pathological fractures, and bony deformities in the limbs. The changes may be generalised or limited to a single bone, but the skull, axial skeleton and proximal regions of the tubular bones are most frequently involved. Classically, three stages are described: an initial active or destructive phase, a combined destructive and reparative phase, and a final quiescent sclerotic phase. The radiographic appearances are thus extremely variable, but in long-standing cases the bones are expanded, with diffuse sclerosis and lytic areas and an abnormal trabecular pattern. Excessive vascularity of the bones is usual and sarcomatous changes occur in about 5% of patients.

The alkaline phosphatase concentration is consistently elevated in all but the early and monostotic cases. The diseased bones show a decreased calcium content and current interest centres around therapy with calcitonin and diphosphates (GOLDFIELD et al. 1972; RUSSELL 1974).

2. Pachydermoperiostosis

In pachydermoperiostosis, clubbing of the digits, thickening of the skin of the extremities, and oiliness of the scalp are associated with widening and sclerosis of the cortices of the long bones. At the distal ends, periosteal thickening and medullary trabeculation are often evident. The dermal changes are of assistance in differentiation from pulmonary osteoarthropathy and thyroid acropathy.

The manifestations of pachydermoperiostosis and the underlying physiological mechanisms were reviewed by RIMOIN (1965). In a recent report of three cases, DIJAN et al. (1976) re-emphasised that the condition has a predilection for males and that the range of severity is very variable.

CURRARINO et al. (1961) and CHAMBERLAIN et al. (1965) reported a similar disorder under the title 'familial idiopathic osteoarthropathy.' This condition was recognised in a Negro kindred in the U.S.A. and the main features were subperiosteal new bone formation, defective cranial ossification, clubbing of the fingers, and eczematous skin eruptions. CREMIN (1970) described a girl aged 18 months in whom layered periosteal reaction on the tubular bones was associated with wide fontanelles and sutures. Clubbed fingers were present in other members of the family.

In the Touraine-Solenti-Golé syndrome, hyperostosis of the frontal region of the skull and the cortices of the tubular bones is associated with digital clubbing, pachydermia and familial acromegaly in the absence of any abnormality of growth hormone (GRAY and STEYN 1978). This condition, which develops after puberty, seems to be distinct from the other pachydermia-hyperostosis syndromes.

3. Stanescu Syndrome

STANESCU et al. (1963) described an autosomal dominant disorder in which short stature, brachycephaly, and a wide mandibular angle were associated with sclerosis and widening of the cortices of the tubular bones. The condition bears some resemblance to pycnodysostosis but may be distinguished by the absence of bony fragility and the lack of changes in the terminal phalanges.

The only report is that of the original authors, who studied 11 members of three generations of a French kindred.

4. Tubular Stenosis

KENNY and LINARELLI (1966) described a mother and son with 'dwarfism and cortical thickening of the tubular bones.' These patients had frontal bossing, and episodes of hypocalcaemic tetany and convulsions had occurred during infancy.

The radiographic features were reviewed by CAFFEY (1967) and FRECH and McALISTER (1968), who pointed out that the diaphyses of the long bones show massive sclerosis and endosteal hyperostosis, with narrowing of the medullary canals and attentuation of the shafts. The condition is generally known as 'tubular stenosis,' or the 'Kenny-Caffey syndrome.'

SEGOND et al. (1973) reported a mother and two adult sons with a skeletal dysplasia which bore some resemblance to tubular stenosis. However, the normal stature, clinical silence and widespread sclerotic bone changes indicate that it is a separate entity.

5. Familial Osteodysplasia

BUCHIGNANI et al. (1972) described four siblings, two brothers and two sisters, with cortical hyperostosis and medullary cavity narrowing, in association with prominence of the brows, flattening of the nasal bridge, dental malocclusion, mid-facial hypoplasia and scoliosis. In view of the widespread skeletal changes, the authors proposed the name 'familial osteodysplasia' for the syndrome.

Radiologically, cortical thickening was maximal in the femora, and other changes included brachycephaly, calvarial thinning, hypoplasia of the spinous processes of some cervical vertebrae, and disproportion between the phalanges in the feet. The superior pubic rami and the ribs were thin.

The clinical features of the same kindred were the subject of a separate paper by ANDERSON et al. (1972). Consanguinity was present and it is likely that inheritance was autosomal recessive. Familial osteodysplasia is a different entity from the osteodysplasty of MELNICK and NEEDLES (see Chap. 10).

6. Schwarz-Lélek Syndrome

The eponymous designation 'Schwarz-Lélek syndrome' was used by GORLIN, SPRANGER and KOSZALKA (1969) for two males with a distinctive skeletal dysplasia. These individuals had been reported by SCHWARZ (1960) as 'craniometaphyseal dysplasia' and by LÉLEK (1961) as 'Camurati-Engelmann disease.' A young woman described by STACK (1900) as having 'diffuse leontiasis ossea' had similar phenotypic features and may also have had the syndrome.

The main radiological manifestations were hyperostosis and sclerosis of the frontal and occipital regions of the skull with pronounced lateral bowing and metaphyseal widening of the femora. The genetic basis of the condition is unknown.

7. Sclerotic Bone-Dentine Dysplasia Syndrome

MORRIS and AUGSBURGER (1977) described a Californian kindred in which skeletal sclerosis and radicular dentine dysplasia of the teeth were transmitted through four generations as an autosomal dominant trait. The radiographic description was incomplete, but endosteal cortical thickening and sclerosis of the long bones and carpus were mentioned.

8. Osteopetrosis with Familial Paraplegia

JACQUES et al. (1975) reported a North American kindred in which individuals in three generations had dominantly inherited osteopetrosis and late-onset paraplegia, in the absence of any clinical or myelographic evidence of spinal cord compression. The syndromic status of this disorder is uncertain.

9. Central Osteosclerosis with 'Bamboo Hair'

JOHNSON et al. (1978) described an infant with sclerosis of the central skeleton, including the skull, spine, thoracic cage and pelvis in association with 'bamboo hair' and ichthyosis. The appendicular skeleton showed osteoporosis, which was attributed to disuse.

The abnormalities in the skin and hair are consistent with a diagnosis of the Netherton syndrome, but bone sclerosis is not usually seen in this condition. The authors speculated that the skeletal changes might be a genuine component of this disorder, which had previously escaped notice.

10. Weismann-Netter-Stuhl Syndrome (Toxopachyostéose Diaphysaire Tibio-Péronière)

This rare disorder, which has a complex anatomical title and a cumbersome eponymous designation, presents as 'sabre shins.' Besides anterior curvature of the tibia and fibula, stature may be short and mental deficiency is sometimes present. Involvement may be asymmetrical and severity is variable. The condition is inherited as an autosomal dominant and many of the reported patients have been of African Negro stock. About 15 cases can be recognised in the literature (KEATS and ALAVI 1970; ALAVI and KEATS 1973; AZIMI and BRYAN 1974).

Radiographically a major feature is anterior bowing of the tibia and fibula, with lesser degrees of curvature of the other long bones of the limbs. Endosteal cortical hyperostosis is prominent in the diaphyses, but the external contours of these bones are undisturbed. Gross kyphoscoliosis is sometimes present. The iliae have a square configuration, and the falx cerebri may be calcified.

The syndrome is easily differentiated from dietary rickets by the lack of metaphyseal involvement, and from congenital syphilis by the predominant posterior distribution of the cortical thickening and the absence of other stigmata of luetic disease.

References

1. Osteitis Deformans

BARRY HC (1969) Paget's disease of bone. Edinburgh, Livingstone

BRAILSFORD JF (1954) Paget's disease of bone. Br J Radiol 27:435

GUYER DE, CLOUGH PW (1978) Paget's disease of bone. Clin Radiol 29:41

GOLDFIELD EB, BRAIKER BM, PRENDERGAST JJ, KOLB FO (1972) Synthetic salmon calcitonin. Treatment of Paget's disease and osteogenesis imperfecta. J A M A 221:1127

NAGER GT (1975) Paget's disease of the temporal bone. Ann Otolaryngol 84:22

RUSSELL RGG, SMITH R, PRESTON C, WALTON RJ, WOODS CG (1974) Diphosphonates in Paget's disease. Lancet 1:894

2. Pachydermoperiostosis

CHAMBERLAIN DS, WHITAKER J, SILVERMAN FN (1965) Idiopathic osteoarthropathy and cranial defects in children. (Familial idiopathic osteoarthropathy). A J R 93:408

CREMIN BJ (1970) Familial idiopathic osteoarthropathy of children: A case report and progress. Br J Radiol 43:568

CURRARINO G, TIERNEY RC, GIESEL RG, WEIHL C (1961) Familial idiopathic osteoarthropathy. A J R 85:633

DIJAN A, SEBAOUN J, BEASLEY N (1976) Three chance observations of pachydermoperiostosis. Rev Rhum Mal Osteoartic 43:528

GRAY PI, STEYN AF (1978) Touraine-Solenti-Golé syndrome: A case report. S Afr Med J 54:1071

RIMOIN DL (1965) Pachydermoperiostosis (idiopathic clubbing and periostosis). Genetic and physiologic considerations. N Engl J Med 272:923

3. Stanescu syndrome

STANESCU V, MAXIMILIAN C, POENARU S, FLOREA I, STANESCU R, IONESCO V, IONITIU D (1963) Syndrome hereditaire dominant. Rev Fr Endocrinol Clin 4:219

4. Tubular stenosis

CAFFEY J (1967) Congenital stenosis of medullary spaces in tubular bones and calvaria in two proportional dwarfs – mother and son, coupled with transitory hypocalcemic tetany. A J R 100:1

Frech RS, McAlister WH (1968) Medullary stenosis of the tubular bones associated with hypocalcemic convulsions and short stature. Radiology 91:457

Kenny FM, Linarelli L (1966) Dwarfism and cortical thickening of the tubular bones: Transient hypocalcaemia in a mother and son. Am J Dis Child 111:201

Segond P, Menkes CJ, Maroteaux P, Braun S, Delbarre F (1973) Le rétrécissement du canal médullaire des os à transmission dominante. Nouv Presse Méd 2:2728

5. Familial osteodysplasia

Anderson LG, Cook AJ, Coccaro PJ, Bosma JF (1972) Familial osteodysplasia. J A M A 220:1687

Buchignani JS, Cook AJ, Anderson LG (1972) Roentgenographic findings in familial osteodysplasia. A J R 116:602

6. Schwarz-Lélek syndrome

Gorlin RJ, Spranger J, Koszalka MF (1969) Genetic craniotubular bone dysplasias and hyperostoses: A critical analysis. Birth Defects 5/4:79

Lélek I (1961) Camurati-Engelmann'sche Erkrankung. Fortschr Roentgenstr 94:702

Schwarz E (1960) Craniometaphyseal dysplasia. A J R 84:461

Stack EHE (1900) A case of diffuse leontiasis ossea. Bristol Med Chir J 18:316

7. Sclerotic bone-dentine dysplasia syndrome

Morris ME, Augsburger RH (1977) Dentine dysplasia with sclerotic bone and skeletal anomalies inherited as an autosomal dominant trait. Oral Surg 43:267

8. Osteopetrosis with familial paraplegia

Jacques S, Garner JT, Johnson D, Sheldon CH (1975) Osteopetrosis associated with familial paraplegia: Report of a family. Paraplegia 13:143

9. Central osteosclerosis with bamboo hair

Johnson F, Flores C, Dodgson WB (1978) Case report 50. Skeletal Radiol 2:185

Netherton EW (1958) A unique case of trichorrhexis nodosa. Arch Dermatol 78:483

10. Weismann-Netter-Stuhl syndrome (toxopachyostéose diaphysaire tibio-péronière

Alavi SM, Keats TE (1973) Toxopachyostéose diaphysaire tibio-péronière. Weismann-Netter syndrome. A J R 118:314

Azimi F, Bryan PJ (1974) Weismann-Netter-Stuhl syndrome (Toxopachyostéose diaphysaire tibio-péronière). Br J Radiol 47:618

Keats TE, Alavi MS (1970) Toxopachyostéose diaphysaire tibio-péronière (Weismann-Netter syndrome). A J R 109:568

This girl presented at one year of age with swelling of the legs. It was noted that she had a mild eczema of her face, digital clubbing, and open fontanelles. The skeletal defects resolved over the next four years. There was a family history of clubbing and a diagnosis of familial idiopathic osteoarthropathy was made. This condition should be differentiated from pachydermoperiostitis, in which there is generalised skin thickening

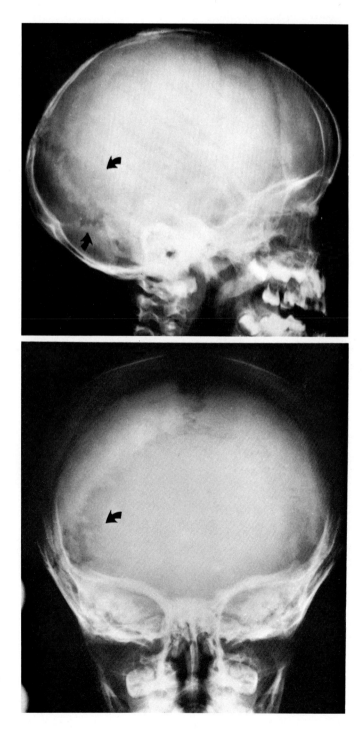

Fig. 21-1 a and b. Skull. At 2 years of age the fontanelles were open, with bony deficiency (arrows) and wormian bones in the lambdoid sutures (Cremin 1970)

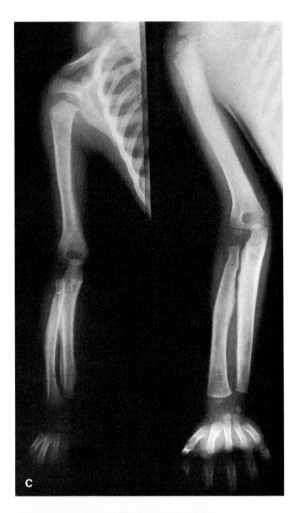

Fig. 21-1. (c) Arm. Marked periosteal reaction at one year, which is resolving at 2 years of age (Cremin 1970). (d) Hand at 2 years. There is soft-tissue clubbing of terminal phalanges and the epiphyseal development is retarded by about six months (Cremin 1970). (e) Legs. Periosteal layering at one year and residual thickening at 2 years. The changes had resolved completely at 5 years (Cremin 1970)

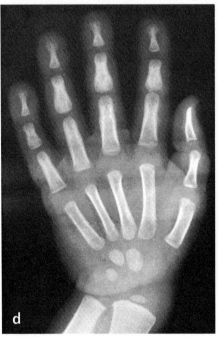

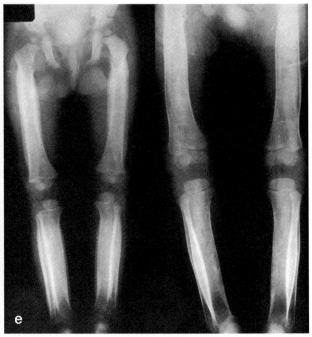

Chapter 22

Differential Diagnosis:
Other Sclerosing Disorders

Osteoblastic secondary neoplastic deposits and lymphomas may produce diffuse or localised areas of skeletal sclerosis. In practice, their clinical and radiological features are unlikely to be mistaken for those of the dysplasias described in the preceding chapters. There exists, however, a residue of conditions which may cause confusion, and a brief description of these is given in this chapter.

1. Fluorosis
2. Heavy-metal poisoning
3. Renal osteosclerosis
4. Myelosclerosis
5. Mastocytosis
6. Tuberous sclerosis
7. Other mechanisms of sclerosis

For the sake of brevity, references are not cited in the text of this section, but relevant reviews are listed under the appropriate headings at the end of the chapter.

1. Fluorosis

This disorder is typically found in rural populations who habitually drink well-water with a high fluoride content and it reaches a high prevalence in certain regions of the Punjab in India and in South Africa. Fluorosis is also occasionally encountered as an occupational disease in the production of aluminium and fertilisers. Chronic fluoride poisoning causes dental mottling and, in advanced cases, limitation of articular mobility.

The radiological signs include trabecular thickening and, in the late stages, diffuse amorphous homogeneous sclerosis of the cortex and medulla. The density is widespread throughout the axial and appendicular skeleton. The skull is not particularly involved, but in childhood marrow hyperplasia may occasionally be seen in the calvarium and ribs. Roughening of the muscle attachments at the iliac spines and crests is a useful early diagnostic feature, while calcification of ligamentous attachments, especially in the pelvis and spine and in the interosseous membranes, is a late manifestation.

The skeleton shows a striking amorphous density which could easily be confused with osteopetrosis, and for this reason two cases of fluorosis are depicted in this chapter.

2. Heavy-Metal Poisoning

Lead, phosphorus and bismuth intoxication may produce bands of increased density in the metaphyseal regions. These are uncommon conditions but lead poisoning is still sometimes seen in children who have inadvertently ingested the metal. Radiographically, the zones of provisional calcification in the metaphyses show wide bands of markedly increased density. These changes in the growing ends of bone are probably due to a disturbance of endochondral ossification rather than actual deposition of the heavy metal.

In long-standing cases, the metaphyseal ends of the long bones become 'clubbed' from lack of modelling, while the dense bands may show stratification. These appearances bear a superficial resemblance to those of osteopetrosis.

3. Renal Osteosclerosis

'Renal osteodystrophy' is the term used to describe the skeletal abnormalities associated with renal failure. These are predominantly osteomalacia and secondary hyperparathyroidism, but sclerotic changes may be seen in the growing skeleton. At this stage the newly laid-down bone has a fine cortical trabecular meshwork with obliteration of the medulla. These changes are maximal at the long-bone metaphyses, and in the pubis, base of the skull, and the end plates of the vertebra. Over a quarter of a century ago the late Dr C. E. Dent of University College Hospital, London, coined the phrase 'rugger jersey spine' for the radiographic appearance of vertebral bodies affected in this way. This term is now more widely used in the context of the osteopetroses (see Chap. 4).

Sclerosis is not usually a sequel of renal tubular acidosis unless there is renal failure. The primary radiological manifestations are nephrocalcinosis, nephrolithiasis and osteomalacia, but diffuse sclerosis of thoracic and lumbar spine, pelvis, and upper femora in an adult woman with uncomplicated renal tubular acidosis has been reported by Chin and Cheah (1977).

4. Myelosclerosis

Proliferation of the bone marrow in anaemia can rarefy the medulla. Conversely, trabecular reaction to marrow hyperplasia causes increased density. The radiological spectrum includes loss of trabecular pattern, diffuse ground-glass opacification, and focal changes such as mottled opacities, dense endosteal plates in the vertebral bodies, and endocortical thickening with loss of marrow cavity in long bones. The ribs and thoracic spine are commonly involved, but the lumbar vertebrae, pelvis and limb bones may be sclerotic. The presence of splenomegaly is a frequent and important diagnostic pointer.

5. Mastocytosis

In this condition, mast cell proliferation occurs in many sites, including the skin (urticaria pigmentosa), gut, and bone. The skeletal changes are variable and may be localised or diffuse, lytic or sclerotic, or appear as patchy densities interspersed with porosis. The diffuse sclerotic lesions are widespread in distribution but are most frequent in skull, vertebrae, ribs and pelvis.

6. Tuberous Sclerosis

The clinical features of this autosomal dominant disorder are mental retardation, epilepsy, adenoma sebaceum and cutaneous fibromata. Radiographically, ill-defined diffuse axial and appendicular bone densities may be evident. Other changes include cysts and cortical irregularities in the bones of the hands and feet and intracerebral calcifications.

7. Other Mechanisms of Sclerosis

Generalised skeletal sclerosis of mild degree may be a transient feature of the neonatal period, when it is known as 'physiological osteosclerosis of the newborn.' At this stage of life, erythroblastosis fetalis may also cause a generalised increase in bone density.

Repeated episodes of trauma can result in sclerosis of the affected bone. This situation may be encountered in the 'battered baby,' where other asymmetrical features, including fractures, dislocations, metaphyseal distortion, and diaphyseal bowing are valuable diagnostic indicators.

Hypervitaminosis A is a rare cause of generalised periosteal reaction in the tubular bones, which resembles CAFFEY's infantile cortical hyperostosis. The onset after the first year of life, absence of pyrexia and the additional features of weight loss and yellow discoloration of the skin serve to distinguish the former condition. The bone changes regress after reduction of excessive vitamin A intake.

Chronic overdose with vitamin D leads to hypercalcaemia and renal damage. Radiographically, the skull and vertebrae are dense, and deposits of calcium may be evident in the periarticular soft tissues, arterial walls and falx cerebri.

8. Comments

The conditions which we have discussed in this chapter may not all be accepted as 'bone dysplasias' but they have been selected because they are relevant and may cause confusion with our other subject matter.

We must emphasise that it is impossible to include every disorder which causes bone sclerosis. Equally, the question of sclerosing neoplasms of bone, whether they be osteogenic, cartilaginous or neurogenic, is also beyond the scope of this book. Any radiologist with experience will recognise that in this situation, when doubt arises, the appropriate course of action would be to refer to such excellent standard monographs as those by EDEIKEN and HODES (1973) and MURRAY and JACOBSON (1977). Current concepts in the wide field of osteology have recently been reviewed by FELDMAN (1978).

References

1. Fluorosis

MURRAY RO, JACOBSON HC (1977) Fluorosis. In: The radiology of skeletal disorders, 2nd ed, vol 1. Churchill Livingstone, London, p. 580

2. Heavy-Metal Poisoning

CAFFEY J (1973) Pediatric X-ray diagnosis, 6th ed, vol 2. Year Book Medical Publishers Chicago

3. Renal Osteosclerosis

CHIN WS, CHEAH JS (1977) Osteosclerosis in renal tubular acidosis: A case report. Australas Radiol 21:343

DENT CE, HODSON CJ (1954) General softening of bone due to metabolic causes. II. Radiologic changes associated with certain metabolic bone diseases. Br J Radiol 27:605

EASTWOOD JB (1977) Renal osteodystrophy – A radiological review. Crit Rev Diagn Imaging 9:77

KAYE M, PRITCHARD JE, HALPENNY GW, LIGHT W (1960) Bone disease in chronic renal failure with particular reference to osteosclerosis. Medicine (Baltimore) 39:157

WOLF HL, DENKO JV (1958) Osteosclerosis in chronic renal disease. Am J Med Sci 235:33

ZIMMERMAN HB (1962) Osteosclerosis in chronic renal disease: Report of 4 cases associated with secondary hyperparathyroidism. A J R 88:1152

4. Myelosclerosis

LEIGH TF, CORLEY CC JR, HUGULEY CM JR, ROGERS JV (1959) Myelofibrosis: The general and radiologic findings in 25 proved cases. A J R 82:183

PETTIGREW JD, WARD HP (1969) Correlation of radiologic, histologic and clinical findings in myeloid metaplasia. Radiology 93:541

5. Mastocytosis

EDEIKEN J, HODES PJ (1967) Roentgen diagnosis of diseases of bone, 2nd ed. Williams & Wilkins, Baltimore

WOOTEN WB, DE SANTONS LA, FINKELSTEIN JB (1978) Case report 61: Mastocytosis. Skeletal Radiol 3:53

6. Tuberous Sclerosis

MEDLEY BE, McLEOD RA, WAYNE HOUSER O (1976) Tuberous sclerosis. Semin Roentgenol 11:35

7. Other Mechanisms of Sclerosis

CAFFEY J (1957) Some traumatic lesions in growing bones other than fractures and dislocations: Clinical and radiological features. Br J Radiol 30:225

DESMET AA, KUHNS LR, KAUFMAN RA, HOLT JF (1977) Bony sclerosis and the battered child. Skeletal Radiol 2:39

SILVERMAN FN (1953) The roentgen manifestations of unrecognized skeletal trauma in infants. A J R 69:413

RUBY LK, MITAL MA (1974) Skeletal deformities following chronic hypervitaminosis A. J Bone Joint Surg [Am] 56:1283

8. Comment

EDEIKEN J, HODES PJ (1973) Roentgen diagnosis of diseases. 2nd ed. Williams & Wilkins Baltimore

MURRAY RO, JACOBSON HG (1977) Radiology of skeletal disorders. 2nd edition (4 volumes), Churchill Livingstone, London

FELDMAN F (ed) (1978) Radiology, pathology, and immunology of bones and joints; a review of current concepts. Appleton-Century-Crofts, New York

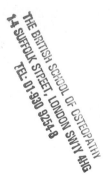

Two cases are presented, both from regions of endemic fluorosis in South Africa. The first patient also exhibits reactive bone marrow hyperplasia

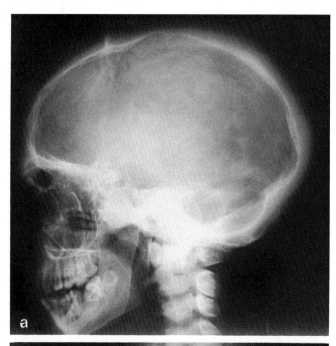

Case I
Boy aged 9 years

Fig. 22-1. (a) Skull. The base is sclerotic and the diploic space of the vault is widened

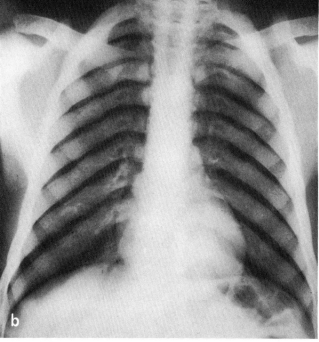

Fig. 22-1. (b) Chest. Sclerosis and widening of ribs and clavicles is evident

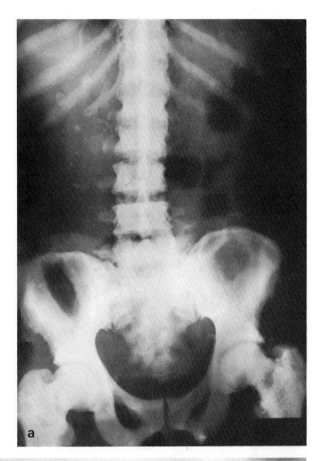

Case II
Male aged
40 years

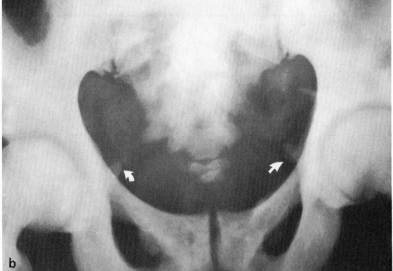

Fig. 22-2. (a) Excretory urogram. Sclerosis of all bones due to fluorosis was
a chance finding. (b) Pelvis. The sacro-iliac ligaments are ossified (arrows)

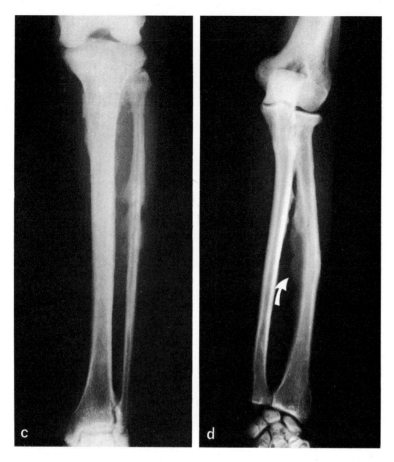

Fig. 22-2. (c) Leg. Sclerosis is present and bone spurs in muscle attachments are a prominent feature. (d) Forearm. The interosseous membrane is ossified (arrow)

Subject Index

B. J. Cremin, P. Beighton

Bone Dysplasias of Infancy

A Radiological Atlas

Foreword from R. O. Murray
1978. 55 figures in 124 separate illustrations, 4 tables. XIII, 109 pages
ISBN 3-540-08816-4

Individually rare, but collectively common, the skeletal dysplasias of
infancy are a fascinating group of conditions in which there has been an
explosion of interest in the last decade. Many new syndromes have been
delineated and in these, diagnostic accuracy is crucial for meaningful
prognostication and genetic counselling. As diagnosis is based on the
recognition of characteristic radiographic manifestations, the radiologist
plays a key role in the management of patients with these disorders.
The skeletal dysplasias that are evident during infancy are depicted and
their clinical, radiographic and genetic features are briefly described. The
classification is based on the updated (1977) Paris nomenclature. The
book has been written for radiologists and pediatricians to facilitate easy
recognition of these conditions. Techniques of antenatal diagnosis are
also dicussed.

Contents: Clinical and Genetic Evaluation of the Neonate with Skeletal
Dysplasia. – Radiographic Techniques. – Achondrogenesis. – Thanato-
phoric Dysplasia. – Asphyxiating Thoracic Dysplasia. – Chondroecto-
dermal Dysplasia. – Lethal Short Rib-Polydactyly Syndromes. –
Chondrodysplasia Punctata. – Campomelic Dysplasia. – Achondroplasia. –
Diastrophic Dysplasia. – Metatropic Dysplasia. – Spondyloepiphyseal
Dysplasia Congenita. – Mesomelic Dysplasia. – Larsen Syndrome. –
Cleido-Cranial Dysplasia. – Osteogenesis Imperfecta Congenita. –
Hypophosphatasia. – Osteopetrosis and Other Sclerosing Bone Dsy-
plasias.

From the reviews:
"...excellent illustrations... assist in making a definitive diagnosis... of great
value to the paediatrician, the geneticist and the radiologists."
South African Medical Journal

"(What the authors present) not only indicates the value of many new
diagnostic techniques in the early recognition of these disorders, but offers
an accurate prognosis for many of these affected children."
Orthopaedic Review

"...recommended for all those who encounter these rare syndromes on
occasion... a prerequisite for intelligent prognoses and family guidance."
Geburtshilfe und Frauenheilkunde

"Differential diagnosis provided briefly and didactically for the non-
specialist unacquainted with these confusing diseases... Strongly recom-
mended for pediatricians, pediatric radiologists and orthopedic surgeons."
Röntgenpraxis

"...outstanding illustrative material..."
Fortschritte auf dem Gebiet der Röntgenstrahlen

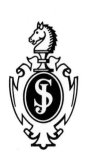
Springer-Verlag
Berlin
Heidelberg
New York

Of further interest:

I. Yaghami

Angiography of Bone and Soft Tissue Lesions

1979. 183 figures in 689 separate illustrations. XI, 459 pages
ISBN 3-540-09147-5

Acetabular Dysplasia – Skeletal Dysplasias in Childhood

Editor: U. H. Weil
With contributions by W. Dega, G. D. MacEwen, E. Morscher, H. L. Moss, J. A. Ogden, W. Schuster, J. Spranger, D. C. Stephens, J. Strauß, H. Wagner
1978. 133 figures, 20 tables. IX, 200 pages
(Progress in Orthopedic Surgery, Volume 2)
ISBN 3-540-08400-2

Comprehensive
Manuals
in Radiology

Editor: H. G. Jacobsen

W. J. Weston, D. G. Palmer

Soft Tissues of the Ectremities

A Radiologic Study of Rheumatic Disease

1978. 171 figures. XV, 128 pages
ISBN 3-540-90259-7

B. T. Katzen

Interventional Diagnostic and Therapeutic Procedures

With contributions by numerous experts
1980. Approx. 150 figures. Approx. 320 pages
ISBN 3-540-90390-9

Current
Diagnostic
Pediatrics

Series Editor: A. R. Chrispin

Current Concepts in Pediatric Radiology

Editor: O. Eklöf
With contributions by numerous experts
1977. 165 figures in 265 separate illustrations, 12 tables. X, 150 pages
ISBN 3-540-08279-4

J. L. Gwinn, P. Stanley

Diagnostic Imaging in Pediatric Trauma

With contributions by G. F. Gates, F. A. Lee, J. G. McComb, J. H. Miller, C. J. Schatz, H. D. Segall, F. Y. Tsai
1980. 275 figures in 468 separate illustrations. Approx. 220 pages
ISBN 3-540-09473-3

Springer-Verlag
Berlin
Heidelberg
New York

Diagnostic Imaging of the Kidney and Urinary Tract in Children

By A. R. Chrispin, I. Gordon, C. Hall, C. Metreweli
1980. 271 figures in 418 separate illustrations, 17 tables. Approx. 220 pages
ISBN 3-540-09472-5